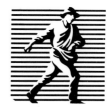

Also by Jose Eber
SHAKE YOUR HEAD, DARLING

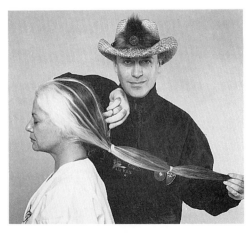

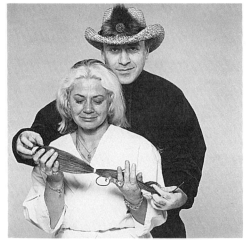

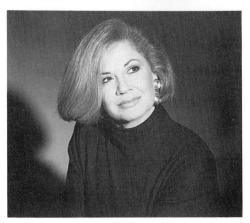

THE
ULTIMATE
MAKEOVER
BOOK

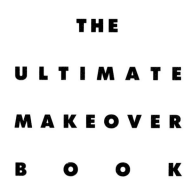

**PHOTOGRAPHS
BY
MICHAEL
CHILDERS**

SIMON AND SCHUSTER

NEW YORK   LONDON

TORONTO   SYDNEY

TOKYO   SINGAPORE

Jose Eber

BEYOND HAIR

Simon and Schuster
Simon & Schuster Building
Rockefeller Center
1230 Avenue of the Americas
New York, New York 10020

SIMON AND SCHUSTER and colophon are registered trademarks
of Simon & Schuster, Inc.

Designed by Bonni Leon
Manufactured in the United States of America

3   5   7   9   10   8   6   4   2

Library of Congress Cataloging in Publication Data
Jose Eber: Beyond Hair. The ultimate makeover book.
Photographs by Michael Childers.
p.   cm.
1. Hairdressing.   I. Childers, Michael.   II. Title.
TT972.E186   1990   89-21866
646.7'242—dc20   CIP
ISBN 0-671-68301-2

Credits

Cover
Jose's outfit by Go Silk courtesy of Theodore's, Beverly Hills. Faye Beland's outfit by Taxi, Ria Handel's and Debbie Henry's outfits by Isaia, Nani Morita's outfit by Westin Wear, and Lorraine Pettit's outfit by French Vanilla. Jewelry courtesy of J. Gerard, West Hollywood.

Inside
Clothes by Taxi, Isaia, Westin Wear, French Vanilla, Opra, Platinum by Dorothy Scholen, Pronto, Sue Wong, Emil Rustinberg, Kanji on Melrose, J. Gerard, I.B.E., Richard and Company, and L. Bates.

Accessories courtesy of M. Gallery, Dana Hamrow, Laura Vogel Jewelry Treasures, J. Gerard, Dana Designs, Kate Hines, and Maximal Art.

ACKNOWLEDGMENTS

There are many people I would like to thank for their help in bringing this book to press. First and foremost, there is my trusted partner Laurent Dufourg. He shares with me the headaches as well as the joys of running a business. I also must thank the fabulous team of experts who accompanied me on the photo sessions for the making of the book— Jeremy, Sylvie, Sherry, Lisa, Scott, and my assistant David as well as makeup artist Thierry Pourtoy assisted by Linda Schaeffer and Thomas Kolarek. Then, too, there are those who kept things running smoothly back in the salons—artistic director Dominique Elliott, thank you. Thanks also to the chemical technicians, Lisanne, Daniele, Garry, Araxy (who's been with me forever), Enrico, Milika, Roxanne, and Sherry; the hairstylists, Julie, Mary Ellen, Davide, Neil, Frank, Odette, Pamela, Jeff, and Cindy; and the manicurists, Robin and Kate.

Thanks to Fabienne Dufourg, Beatrice Campion, Life Brown, and a special thank you to my dear friend, Sonya Zilberberg, who has been by my side from the beginning.

Thank you to all the stylists, technicians, and makeup artists who have worked with me over the years. Every contribution is important.

Thank you to Michael Childers and to his two hard-working assistants, Johann Wolf and James Fortson, for the beautiful photography.

Thanks to Gretchen Clements and her assistant, Mary Beth McEvily, for their help in supplying the wardrobe used in the photographs.

Many thanks to Marge Schicktanz, Oscar and Gabbie Stempel and family, the late George Kirvay, Alan Neirob, Robin Nyman, Jeffrey Lane, Barbara Bryson, and Alex Yemenidjian.

A very special thank you to my personal assistant, Lillian Morri, who keeps my life running smoothly and is always there for me when I need her.

Thank you to Jan Miller and Allan Mayer who brought this book from idea to reality.

Finally, a big thank you to Catherine McEvily Harris, my collaborator on this book, who started out as a friend in business and has turned into a friend for life.

This book is dedicated to my whole family: to my mother and father, who are no longer with me but who supported me always and taught me the true meaning of love; to my sister, Esther, and my brother, Henry, and their families, who still watch over their baby brother and keep the family together even though we're so far apart.

It is also dedicated to my dear friends (and you all know who you are) who have stayed with me through the hard times as well as the good times—it is a real comfort to know you're there.

And finally, I dedicate this book to every person who has ever walked through the door of one of my salons, ever written to me for advice or watched me on television. Without you, my success would be nonexistent.

C O N T E N T S

WHAT IS BEAUTY?

When you imagine a beautiful person, who comes to mind? Is it a famous celebrity? A friend? A relative? My guess is that whoever you're thinking of right now is probably not yourself. I am going to help you change that—now and forever. Thinking of ourselves as beautiful isn't something that comes easily—unless, of course, we think about how we'd look if we just lost that extra weight or how we'd look in that new outfit or how we looked ten years ago. But looking in the mirror and accepting ourselves as we are today is very difficult. Most of us are brought up to believe that thinking of ourselves as beautiful is vain and impolite. The truth is, it can be—if, that is, you think of beauty as total physical perfection. But consider this. I have become famous for working on the most glamorous women in the world, and the ones who stick in my mind as the real beauties are far from perfect. Believe it.

To me, beauty isn't a tiny little nose, heart-shaped lips, and huge eyes. You have been brainwashed, in a way, if you feel inadequate because your own looks don't match those of the models and actresses whose faces and bodies grace the pages of your favorite magazines. But who is doing the comparing? *You* are. I want each and every woman who reads this book to understand that those women are the minority. Most women don't look like that. As a matter of fact, most of those models and actresses don't look like that until after they've spent hours with a hairstylist, makeup artist, and wardrobe consultant. Believe me, I know.

The fact is, the first step toward beauty is to accept yourself the way you are, to quit comparing yourself with others. Of course, it's smart to keep up with the latest styles in hair and fashion. But you must realize that what you see in fashion magazines is put there as much for entertainment as it is for education. Take from those pages only the things that work for you personally; enjoy the rest as drama and fantasy. If you can do this, your mind will be open to the true meaning of beauty.

Beauty, to me, is the spirit inside a person who touches the lives of everyone she meets with a positive attitude and a strong sense of direction. The beautiful women I know have a self-confidence that comes from knowing that it's okay to be wrong sometimes or insecure sometimes or even unattractive sometimes. They don't feel great because they look beautiful —they look beautiful because they feel great!

Have you ever walked down the street and seen what you consider to be an absolutely gorgeous man with a woman you thought really quite ordinary-looking? What goes through your mind? (Be honest, it's happened to all of us. Men do it, too, when they see a terrific-looking woman with a not-so-hot-looking guy.) She must be an heiress, right? Or maybe his boss? Or at the very least, the boss's daughter. But did you ever consider the possibility that your wide-eyed hunk may see something in this "ordinary" woman that is extraordinary? Wouldn't it make you feel good to think that perhaps this man sees something deeper than her external appearance?

Maybe you have a friend who isn't what you would call beautiful but who is the luckiest person in love you've ever known. Have you thought about why that is? Perhaps he or she isn't beautiful by traditional physical standards, but I bet you'll agree that that person has a "certain something" that causes people to stop and take notice when he or she walks into a room. Again, that "certain something," if you think about it, is probably a self-confidence that is possessed only by those who are at ease with their inner selves.

So how can *you* get that "certain something"? Believe me, it won't come by applying more mascara or sporting a new hairstyle. I think it comes from setting a goal for yourself and then achieving it. Whether it is a career goal or a personal goal, the important thing is to have a sense of direction. As soon as you start to take pride in yourself, I think a self-confidence will begin to emerge that is so natural and unassuming that you won't be aware of anything happening other than the fact that you feel great!

Of course, I do not believe that in order to have real inner beauty, your outer beauty should be ignored. After all, I get *my* pride and self-confidence from having the ability to make women look their best. Concern for your appearance is not vanity as long as it doesn't make you a slave to your makeup bag and mirror. I'll bet you know someone who is absolutely terrified of going out of the house without her makeup. If caught, she will immediately greet you with an apology for the way she looks. To me, this is very silly. Although I do think that most women look better with a bit of makeup, in some cases there just isn't time for a full face. A more confident woman would understand that. Besides, when you point out to people that you are not looking your best, they are bound to notice!

I want you to be as proud of the way you look as you are of the way you feel. Taking the time to learn about the hairstyle, makeup, and clothes that are right for you is time well spent. Don't worry about trying to look like someone else. It is much more exciting to develop a style that's interesting and all your own. Believe me when I tell you, no one has ever told me that I look like anyone else! But that doesn't mean I haven't gone without my own insecurities. For years, I have been known as the man who always wears boots and a cowboy hat. I am going to share with you now a secret that people have asked me about at least a thousand times. I started wearing my signature hat for the same reason I always wore cowboy boots —to make me look taller. I had always dreamed of what it would be like to be a strapping man who stood over six feet tall. As it became clear to me that I would never know what that feels like, I became the master of illusion. Boots added a couple of inches on the bottom and the hat gave me a few more on top. Sounds easy, doesn't it? Well, let me tell you, it wasn't. As a result of my insecurity about my height, I came home many nights with sore, aching feet. But I was not about to take those boots off, no matter how painful they were.

Today, thankfully, things are different. I have accomplished many of the goals I set for myself and have come to appreciate my own self-worth. I know that wouldn't change if I *were* six feet tall. More important, my real friends couldn't care less. The fact is they never cared. Only I did. Still, a lot of good came from that insecurity. I learned a valuable lesson. Accept me for what I am or not at all.

My reasons for wearing the hat today have changed completely. It has become my trademark, one of the things that make me different from anyone else. I turned what I considered a personal flaw into my *own* style, which is exactly what I would like to teach you to do.

Maybe your nose isn't the size and shape you want it to be. Maybe you feel your eyes are too small, your mouth is too big, or your hair is too thin. Well, don't think of your own features as flaws. After all, they are what make you unique. Look at all the celebrities you admire who have distinctive features like these. If perfect noses were a prerequisite to stardom, half of Hollywood would still be undiscovered. Think of some of the women today who have made really important contributions in film, television, and politics. They are invariably thought of as beautiful. Yet if you were to take their features and examine them separately, you would find that it is not the individual features that make these women beautiful but rather the total picture. It is not important that their noses are tiny or their teeth are perfectly straight. What *is* important is that these women have turned their distinctive features into a style that is completely their own.

There are many hairstyles, makeup secrets, and fashion tips I can show you to take the emphasis off certain features and draw attention to more flattering areas. My reason for teaching you these "tricks of the trade" is to de-emphasize what you consider to be your imperfections just enough so that you can forget about them. Believe me, as soon as *you* quit thinking about your flaws, others will, too. And by the time you're finished dazzling people with your sparkling personality, they'll want to be just like you— big nose, thin hair, and all.

Throughout this book you will find real women just like yourself. It was important to me to find models who were totally representative, with problems to which many people can relate. Some of them have hair that is very thick and difficult to manage. Others have hair so thin and fine that it was nearly impossible for them to create a style of their own. A few of the women wanted advice on hairstyles for high foreheads. Some felt their low foreheads were the problem. Some had ears that were better off covered. Others looked best with their hair pulled completely away from their face.

Still, whatever their individual needs, all of these women have something in common. Look closely into their eyes and at their smiles. You can see they have that positive spirit I've been talking about. These women were filled with inner beauty when I met them. All they needed was a little help and advice on how to make their outsides match their insides! Perhaps their questions are the same as your own. Perhaps they have similar lifestyles and time limitations. I think there is some of all of us in each of these fabulous women.

The point is, if you take care of your inner beauty, I can help you with your outer beauty. And the next time someone asks you to think of a beautiful person, you won't have to look far for the answer.

GETTING STARTED

Why is so much emphasis placed on hair? Why are there literally hundreds of thousands of hair salons in the world and new ones opening every day? Why is it often so hard to get an appointment with your favorite hairstylist? And why, once you get that appointment, do you wait for hours to see him or her?

The reason is really quite simple. Your hair surrounds your most obvious form of communication with the rest of the world—your face. Every time you smile, laugh, frown, scream, cry, wink, or talk, you hair is in view. With that kind of exposure, your hair *should* be important to you. And you should know how to make it look fabulous. If you don't, I will show you.

Having the right haircut is the foundation. No amount of color, curl, or spray will camouflage a poor cut. Believe it. For the right cut, you must go to a professional. Please don't try to do it yourself. It is much better to spend the money and have your hair styled right the first time than to go through the expense and aggravation of having it corrected.

So how do you find a great stylist? The best way is to go by the recommendation of a friend or family member, someone with hair similar to yours who has a style that you like. If you don't know anyone with your hair type, there is nothing wrong with asking a stranger who catches your eye. He or she should be flattered by the compliment.

Once you are in the chair, insist that your stylist spend at least five minutes discussing both what you want and what you need (including color and/or perm). If you have seen a hairstyle you like in a book or magazine, cut out the picture and bring it in with you. An experienced professional will be able to tell you whether a particular cut or color suits your hair type, face, image, and life-style. Keep in mind that your stylist works for you—it's not the other way around. In order to keep your business, he or she will have to please you. On the other hand, a true professional will be

E B E R
BEYOND
H A I R

19

honest. He is not doing you any favor by going along with a request of yours that he knows won't work on your type of hair or with your face and body. *Once you have chosen a hairstylist you trust—trust the hairstylist you have chosen.*

Those of you who have seen me on television or had the opportunity to read my first book, *Shake Your Head, Darling,* know the importance I attach to the shape of a woman's face when creating a hairstyle. Of course, it is extremely difficult to discuss face shapes in the abstract. Unless we are talking about identical twins, no two faces are exactly alike. One woman's round face can look completely different from another woman's round face. There are many different variables that determine face shape, things like bone structure, individual facial features, and actual head size.

Still, there are several commonly recognized face shapes that can give you a point of reference, a place to begin before deciding on a new hairstyle. As always, when contemplating a change in your appearance—whether it is in your clothes, your makeup, or your hair—remember that you can de-emphasize the features you feel are less attractive by drawing attention up and away to more flattering areas of your body, face, or head.

Here are the most common and easily recognizable face shapes. Please, keep in mind that these are just to be used as rough guidelines. Many women do not fit neatly into any one category. *And face shape is just one variable to consider when determining a great hairstyle.*

OVAL. Most hairdressers say that the oval face is the ideal shape. The reason is that there is almost nothing to conceal, nothing to compensate for on an oval-shaped face. Therefore, the stylist has more creative freedom.

ROUND. Rarely will you see a face that is actually circular. A round face refers to a shape that lacks sharply defined angles. The cheeks are usually full; so too are the neck and chin area. One way to de-emphasize the roundness (if you'd rather have a sleeker look) is to create the illusion of length by wearing your hair longer, below the jawline. To create a little height on top, ask your stylist about cutting some bangs and then using gel to style them upward.

OBLONG. This face shape is simply long and narrow. One way to compensate for a long face is to add bangs, which create some interest in the middle of the face by drawing the eye downward. Cutting the hair so that it falls between the ear and the chin is another way to draw the attention to the sides of the head rather than to the top and bottom.

SQUARE. A square face has a wide, squared jawline and a straight hairline. The angles may, at times, look sharp or hard. One way to correct this is to style the hair so that the ends are fringed softly around the face, camouflaging the sharp edges.

HEART-SHAPED. A heart-shaped face is wider at the forehead and becomes increasingly narrow toward the jawline. Often the chin appears to be rather pointed. One option for women with heart-shaped faces is to wear their hair chin-length with a lot of fullness at the sides of the head, thus focusing attention away from the chin.

One thing is certain, no one's face is absolutely perfect. But as I always say, who wants to be perfect? Imperfections are what bring character and interest to a face. A face without character quickly becomes a bore. What you need to strive for—and what I can help you with—is the illusion that all your features are in proper proportion to the rest of your face, and that your head is in proper proportion to the rest of your body. The right hairstyle can do that.

What I am trying to tell you is that, yes, face shape is important when choosing a great haircut, but it is no more important than facial features, hair type, hair condition, life-style, and personality. All of these factors work together to give you your own unique style. So, rather than insist, for example, that all women with long faces must have short hair (that would be ridiculous), I will talk about each model's face shape individually and explain how it relates to all the other factors that need to be considered before determining her hairstyle.

Hair color is equally particular. Throughout the pages of this book you will see many different hair colors. Some are natural, some are not. Sometimes we just weren't born with the color that flatters us most. Sometimes we were born with a fabulous color. And sometimes we started out with that fabulous color and somehow lost it somewhere along the way.

There are lots of different reasons for coloring your hair and lots of different ways to do it. Some color is temporary, meaning you can wash it right out if you decide, for some reason, that you don't like the way it looks on you. Other color is permanent; the only way to get rid of it is to grow it out and cut it off. You can have all your hair colored or just part of it, if you like. The list goes on and on. I only have one general piece of advice when it comes to hair color. Even if you happen to be extremely talented with hair, if you do it yourself, be careful. I know many of the home-coloring kits are very popular. They minimize the expense and eliminate the time spent in the salon. But if you haven't had a lot of experience with this sort of thing, ask someone to check your head the first few times you try it in order to make sure you have distributed the color evenly. Nothing looks worse than sloppily colored hair.

Needless to say, there is nothing more appealing than rich, vibrant, lustrous hair, hair that captures people's attention with its rainbow of natural highlights. If you know someone with fabulous hair color, or you happen to see a gorgeous head of hair walking down the street, inspect it closely. You'll notice that beautiful hair is multicolored. Even hair that has never been touched by artificial color has many different shades of natural highlights. That's the way nature works.

Of course, you may want to buck nature altogether and go for the drama of single-colored hair. It may not look natural, but who cares? Sometimes it's just fun to experience the platinum of Marilyn, the fire of Lucy, or the ebony of Elizabeth.

I don't recommend hair color to everyone. Many times I discourage it. When you are lucky enough to have a great color naturally, why mess it up? Sometimes Mother Nature takes very good care of us. This goes back to what we discussed earlier—accepting yourself the way you are. Don't immediately assume there is something wrong with your hair color. Maybe all you need is a deep-conditioning treatment to bring back the shine and luster. Look at our First Lady, Barbara Bush. She is a fine example of a woman who has totally accepted the way she is and has turned it into her own personal style. Sure, she could color her hair, and maybe it would make her look younger. But she doesn't *want* to look younger. Barbara Bush is happy to be a silver-haired grandmother! And why shouldn't she be? She looks terrific! Thanks to her, a lot of women may lose their fear of turning gray; perhaps they'll even look forward to it! I admire Barbara Bush for the contribution she's made to inner beauty.

On the other hand, when a woman *can* enhance her own style by changing the color of her hair, I say go for it! Obviously, the secret to beautifully colored hair is to find a combination of shades that look as if they were created by Mother Nature herself. The problem is that we have allowed ourselves to get into the poor habit of asking for colors that don't really exist in nature. For example, how many times have you actually seen a woman walking down the street with hair the color of a stop sign? Yet we use the term *redhead* all the time. Do yourself a favor. Take a long walk through an open meadow. Observe the colors. As you walk along the *sandy* path, notice the *sun-touched* wild flowers growing freely. See the *buttercups,* the *wheat,* and the *dandelions.* If you happen to find a stick along your path, pick it up and look at the *hickory* bark. Maybe a beautiful *golden*-winged butterfly will flutter along, or you'll hear the unmistakable buzz of a *honey*bee. Follow the path into the nearby woods and see what's there. Depending on the time of year, you might find rich *chestnut* trees with leaves in brilliant combinations of *rust, copper, toast, and caramel.* Smell the intoxicating fragrance of pine and notice the shades of *auburn* and *mahogany* in the soil. As you begin to head home, maybe you glance up into the sky and notice the quiet warnings of a nearby storm. A sky that used to be as blue as a robin's egg is now a swirling mixture of *smoke* and *silver.* The white, pillowlike puffs of clouds have dissolved into sheets of *heather* and *slate.* As you hurry to avoid the inevitable raindrops, remember all the different colors you have seen. While they are still fresh in your mind, maybe you should not go directly home, but instead visit your favorite salon. Now would be the perfect time to discuss your ideal color with your stylist.

Something else you may want to discuss with your stylist is a permanent wave. A permanent wave is a way of rolling your hair around specifically shaped rods in a chemical formula. This chemical formula (commonly referred to as perming solution) breaks down the bonds in the hair, changing the structure, thus allowing the hair to maintain a specific amount of curl or wave. Don't be misled by the name "permanent." The process *does* last a long time, but it still needs to be redone every two to three months depending on your hair type.

Perms are really a fabulous option for women with no time for round brushes, hot rollers, and curling irons. With many perms, it isn't even necessary to blow-dry your hair. You can walk out the door with wet hair and trust that it will dry looking terrific with no help at all!

Perms have improved a great deal in the last ten years. No longer do we automatically associate a permanent wave with a French poodle.

Today there are several different types of perms available. You can have a curly perm, which is wrapped on small rods for a tight curl; a body wave, which is wrapped on very large rods for a loose, easy bend in the hair; a perm weave, in which only certain strands of hair are curled for a very light, natural-looking wave; a spot perm, which gives curl, wave, or body to a specific area such as the crown for height or the ends for direction; a spiral perm, which is rolled on flexible tubes for large, full waves; or a reverse perm, in which very curly hair is rolled on larger rods to soften the hair's natural curl pattern.

Which one is best for you? Again, this depends on the variables we talked about earlier and should be discussed with your hairstylist. I am reluctant to say much more on the subject of perms, because in this case a little knowledge is definitely a dangerous thing. Please, don't give yourself a home permanent unless you are especially fond of wearing a paper bag over your head. If you have ever tried giving yourself a perm, I'm sure you know what I mean. Leave the responsibility to the experts. Believe me, you'll thank me for this advice.

That's not to suggest that there isn't a lot you *can* do yourself. But in order to re-create the salon look in your own home, you must have the same tools available at home that you find at the salon. This doesn't mean that you have to go out and spend a fortune on every lotion, gel, spritz, and foam on the market. Ask your stylist what products you must have in order to make your style work. Generally speaking, you'll find that styling products are not expensive. I happen to be quite proud of my own line distributed nationally through Fabergé, but it is important for you to use the products you like best. Since I will refer to many of these products often throughout the book, I will go over each of them with you now to help you better understand their purpose. I will also explain the purpose of some of the most commonly used hair-styling appliances to help clear up any confusion you might have about their place in your life. Again, you will not and should not use all of these tools, so ask your hairdresser specifically which ones are right for your style.

MOUSSE. I really don't know how women with thin hair ever managed without mousse. It adds body and fullness to lifeless hair almost immediately. Mousse comes in a can and looks and feels a lot like whipped cream. Just as whipped cream fattens up the body, mousse fattens up the hair. It is applied to clean, wet hair at the roots. Read the label of your can of mousse to make sure that it is alcohol-free. Alcohol will deplete your hair of its natural moisture.

GEL. Gel is the greatest product made for achieving maximum control for any style. It enables you to create dramatic styling effects by allowing you to sculpt, shape, scrunch, or spike your hair. Gel is also terrific for taming wild, out-of-control curls. Just a dab the size of a half-dollar in the palm of your hand can work miracles. It can be used on wet or dry hair depending on the look you're after. The fun thing about gel is that you can use it to achieve several completely different looks with the same cut. Ask your hairstylist for suggestions.

STYLING SPRITZ. This product will turn your haircut into your hairstyle. It gives the hair ultra hold in specific areas. Maybe you want to give your bangs some height while the rest of your hair remains free-flowing. Maybe you want the hair on one side of your head to stay away from your face while the other side falls naturally. This is the product that can do the job. Styling spritz can be sprayed on wet or dry hair.

HAIR SPRAY. This is the one product you just don't want to be caught without. It is absolutely essential for keeping your hair in place after you've taken the time to style it. It is also great for emergency touch-ups. Unlike the old days, hair spray no longer has to be stiff or sticky. When it is applied correctly (one light spray around the head should do it), no one should notice you're wearing hair spray at all. It is neither fashionable nor necessary to glue your style into place. A really good hair spray is strong, lightweight, and invisible.

BLOW DRYER. The blow dryer has become standard equipment in both the home and salon. It is faster, more mobile, and much more practical for styling than the old-fashioned hair dryers that women used to sit under for hours at a time. For many of today's coifs, it is the only electric styling tool needed.

DIFFUSER. The diffuser is one of the most important new styling tools to come along in the last few years. It is an attachment that fits on the end of your blow dryer and gives you all the benefits of the heat without the wind. The diffuser virtually eliminates the frizziness so often associated with a permanent wave or naturally curly hair.

HOT ROLLERS. Hot rollers are a fast way to give your hair shape, body, or style. These heated curlers come in assorted sizes for different levels of curl. The larger rollers are used for adding body to straight hair or for loosening tight waves on curly hair. The smaller the roller, the tighter the curl. For a fun, unconstructed-type curl, try the latest in hot roller technology—heated rubber rods that bend around your hair.

CURLING IRON. The curling iron is the most versatile of electric styling tools. But because it applies a lot of heat directly to the hair, it also requires the most talented hand. It is easy to fry your hair with a curling iron, and the only cure for burned hair is a scissors. Once you get the hang of it, though, the curling iron gives you much more control than hot rollers. You can decide where and how much curl each strand of hair should receive. For those of you who have not had a lot of experience, I recommend practicing your style with a cold iron until you feel confident.

FLAT IRON. The flat iron performs a multitude of styling tricks. For those who enjoy the look of a perm every once in a while, but not always, the flat iron is just the tool you need. It can also make curly hair stick-straight, at least temporarily. The flat iron looks like a pair of tongs: instead of wrapping your hair, as with hot rollers and curling irons, you press it between heated plates. Most flat irons have two crimpers, one for soft waves and one for serious, wild waves. Without the crimpers, this appliance does what it says—it irons your hair absolutely flat. The flat iron can straighten even the frizziest hair.

VENT BRUSH. The vent brush is the most commonly used brush for heat-styling your hair. Its plastic teeth are set far apart, and there are holes (vents) in the base of the brush. The vents allow the heat of the blow dryer to reach every strand of hair for faster drying and easier manipulation.

ROUND BRUSH. The round brush is just that—a circular-shaped brush that is used in conjunction with the blow dryer. As you wrap your damp hair around the brush, the hair will dry with a wave. The size of the wave depends on the size of the brush.

FLAT BRUSH. Again, the flat brush is just what its name implies—a flat, square brush that when used on damp hair with a blow dryer will leave the hair straight and flat.

Remember, when you are styling with a blow dryer or diffuser, your hair should be damp, not soaking wet. When you are styling with hot rollers, curling iron, or flat iron, your hair should be absolutely dry.

Although the advantages of styling with heat are enormous, the process is not without its drawbacks. Electric hair appliances can leave hair dry, brittle, split, and frizzy. It is absolutely essential to deep-condition your hair if you style with heat. A quick-conditioning cream rinse is fine for replacing the moisture lost in shampooing. But to repair heat-styled ends, you need a weekly twenty- to thirty-minute treatment with a moisture-rich, deep-conditioning formula.

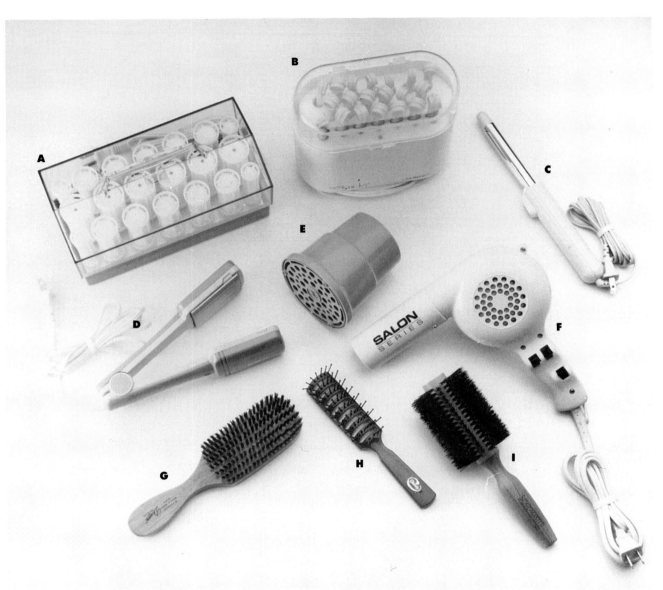

Photograph by Uniack

A. HOT ROLLERS
B. ELECTRIC BENDERS
C. CURLING IRON
D. FLAT IRON
E. DIFFUSER
F. BLOW DRYER
G. FLAT BRUSH
H. VENT BRUSH
I. ROUND BRUSH

MEET THE MODELS

Before I introduce you to the women we selected to illustrate my approach to beauty, I want to tell you a little bit about how and why they were chosen. Over the years, I have seen thousands of women in my salons. And every time I meet a new client, she always asks me the same question. Why would I want to do *her* hair after working on so many beautiful celebrities? You would think that I'd be used to the question by now, but it still shocks me. Why *wouldn't* I want to do her hair, and why wouldn't I think she's beautiful? Because she's not a celebrity? I try to find beauty in all women, and if I can help someone discover a sense of beauty that she has not discovered herself, my work becomes all the more rewarding.

For that reason, when I first thought about doing this book, I decided to demonstrate my techniques not with celebrities or professional models, but with regular women who face the kinds of problems that I see and am asked about every day. The women you will meet in this book are women like yourself—career women, housewives, students. They are tall, short, thin, heavy, black, white, Oriental, old, and young.

I want to make it clear that there are no tricks involved here. When we took the "before" pictures, we photographed the women exactly as they looked when they walked in the door. If they were wearing makeup when they arrived, we left it on. If they weren't wearing any, we did not ask them to apply it. We didn't touch their hair—either to comb it out or mess it up. As a result, you will meet these women the same way I did.

The decision on how to cut, style, and/or color each woman's hair was made jointly by each individual woman and me. Both of us had to agree that the look was right. Equally important, the techniques had to be easy enough for each woman to be able to reproduce them at home. After all, what purpose does a makeover really serve if the positive changes can never be achieved again? There is an old saying I heard once, and it has stuck in my mind ever since. Perhaps you have heard it, too. *Give a man a fish, and he has food for one meal. Teach a man to fish, and he has food for a lifetime.* The point of this exercise was not simply to give these women a makeover, nor just to entertain you with a picture book. The idea was to show you how to identify and solve problems—and how to apply the solutions by yourself in your own home.

In the pages that follow, as you watch our subjects being transformed, remember that their problems are no different from yours. Their photographs are neither retouched nor airbrushed. We weren't striving for perfection—being unique is much more fun.

The beauty you will see in the "after" pictures was right there all along. Discovering it together was nothing less than thrilling.

Jose Eber

BEYOND

HAIR

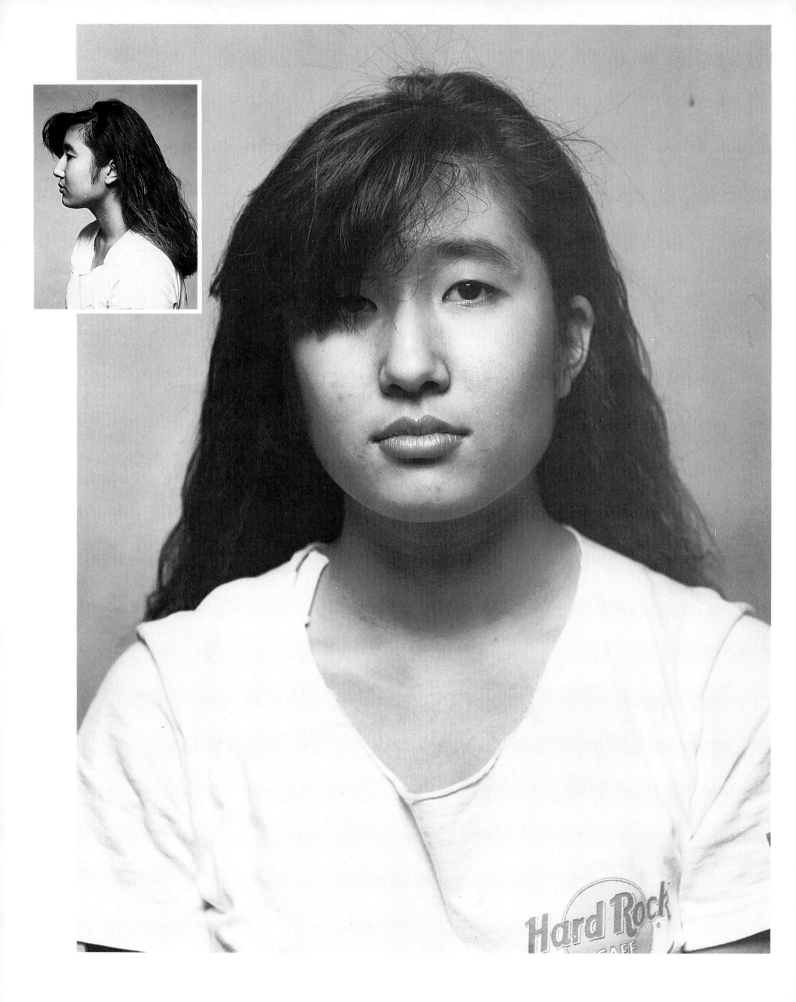

1

A TEEN'S FIRST "LOOK"

NANI MORITA

AGE: 18

OCCUPATION:
PART-TIME
OFFICE CLERK/
FULL-TIME
STUDENT

PROBLEM:
SMALL EYES,
SHORT FOREHEAD,
WIDE FACE

N A N I   M O R I T A

Nani was so cute and little, everyone at the salon wanted to squeeze her cheeks and give her a hug. I must admit, she was a very good sport about it. When I saw her for the first time, I thought, *This* is a darling young girl, but she allows herself to look like every other teenager I see on the street. I wanted her to be an individual, to have a look of her own.

Nani's heritage is part Hawaiian and part Japanese. She has beautiful, thick, healthy hair that can handle just about any style at all. I thought it would be fun to cut her hair in a way that would show off her youthfulness. I asked Nani what she had in mind for herself, and she said she didn't know. Then I asked her if she enjoyed fooling around with her hair, and she said yes, when she knows what she's doing. But since no one ever really taught her how to fix her hair, Nani got in the habit of wearing it the same way all the time. I was determined to end her dilemma. I took a long, hard look at little Nani and asked her if she was ready for a big change. With a nervous giggle, she said yes. . . .

The first thing anyone notices about Nani is her sweet smile and creamy complexion. I knew a younger, more up-to-date cut would give her a new sense of fun and help to develop her own personal style. What I did to Nani was give her a nineties' version of the shag, a style that became popular in the early seventies. Layering her hair all over her head, I cut it close on the sides, leaving some length on the neck and on top. Cutting her hair in this fashion elongated Nani's head, giving her the illusion of a narrower face. A few spiky bangs pulled casually over one eye added a touch of whimsy to complete the look.

At eighteen, Nani shouldn't became a slave to color. Still, I thought it would be fun to give her hair just a bit of drama. Using a nonperoxide mixture of plum and mahogany, I gave Nani a few streaks of excitement. It has been my experience in working with many Asian women that for all the poreless beauty of the Oriental complexion, often the skintone *does* have a yellowish cast to it. It is also true that Oriental men and women almost always have naturally black or very dark brown hair. To change the color dramatically would thus most definitely look unnatural. As I mentioned earlier, sometimes it's fun to buck the system and go for a look that is completely unexpected. But although Nani was willing to make a change, she preferred not to go quite that far. So I chose the mahogany and plum shades, subtle colors that would reflect a soft pink glow onto her skin. This immediately brightened up her face and diffused the yellow.

Because nonperoxide coloring fades away with every shampoo, Nani won't have to worry about her roots growing out and the expense of touchups. However, she now knows how to add a little more excitement and drama to her look whenever the occasion calls for it.

When we were finished, instead of looking like every other eighteen-year-old in town, Nani had a style that was completely her own. But not for long. At last count, three of her friends had requested the same haircut! Oh, well, if you asked Nani, I'm sure she'd agree that it's much more fun being a trendsetter than a trend follower.

DOING IT YOURSELF

TOOLS NEEDED: Mousse, styling spritz, gel, blow dryer, large round brush, hair spray.

It will take you no time at all to get the hang of maintaining this style by yourself. After shampooing, you apply a little mousse to your roots for extra body. Wrapping the ends of your hair around a large round brush, you then blow-dry the top and sides away from your face. After that, use the same technique to bend the ends on your neck slightly under. Now for the fun part. With a small amount of gel on your fingers, you lift up the hair on the very top of your head and hit it with a little styling spritz to hold it in place. Then pull your bangs forward, a few small sections at a time, and do the same thing. A little more gel to hold the sides close to your head, followed by a light coat of hair spray all over, and you're done.

NANI'S COMMENTS

I got scared when Jose asked me if I was ready for a big change. Of course I was scared. I had worn my hair the same way almost my whole life. But then he made me laugh again by telling me he was going to make me look like Joan Jett or Pat Benatar. I *thought* he was just kidding. When he was all done, I couldn't believe it was me. I was in shock, but I loved the look of the girl in the mirror—whoever she was.

If it wasn't for Jose, I would still look the same as I did before. I probably would have looked that way forever. This experience broke a barrier for me—my fear of being different.

When Jose told me I looked like every other teenager on the street, I really didn't know what he meant. Soon after that, I was shopping in a mall with my mom. When I looked around at all the girls hanging out there, it hit me—hard. Every one of them looked like they'd taken clothes from the same closet. Their hair all looked the same, and they were all doing the same thing—nothing. It frightened me to think I used to be just like that. I think we all go through a phase in life when it's comforting to be a follower, it's safe to blend in and not draw attention to yourself.

But then, if you're lucky, you are given the opportunity to be a leader, to do something on your own. And then you discover how good it feels, and you're moved to do it again. It's a lot to learn from one haircut, isn't it?

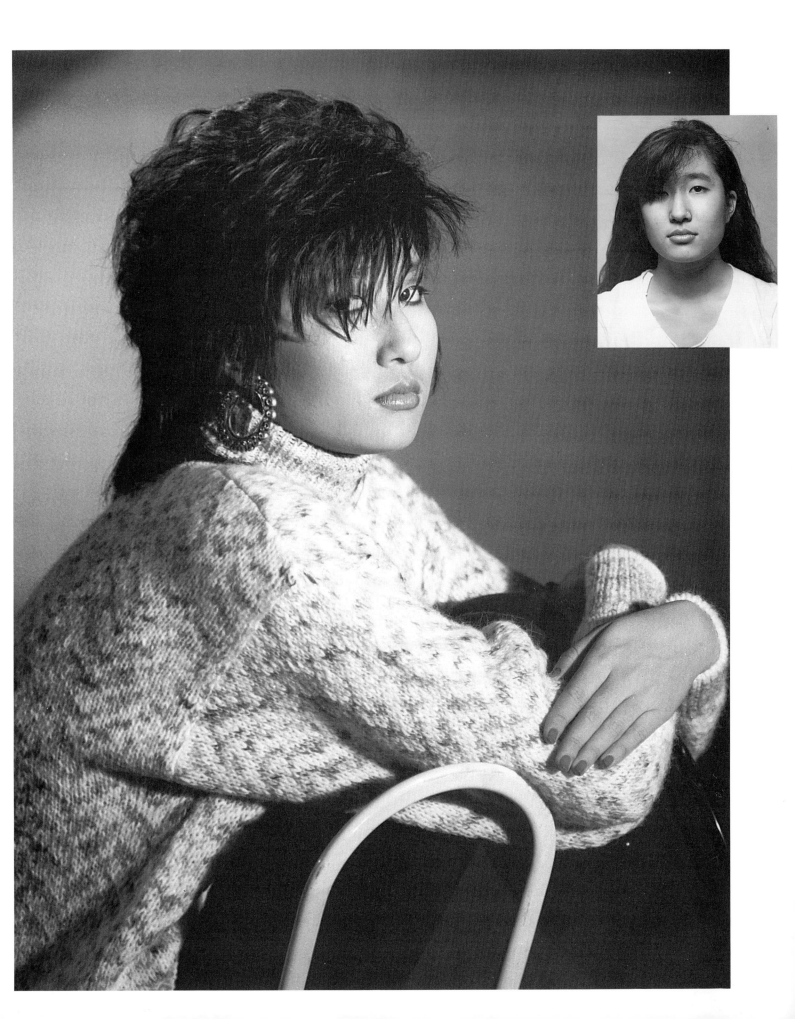

2

INNOCENT *AND* SEXY

TARA ELLISON

AGE: 21

OCCUPATION: RECEPTIONIST/ ACTING STUDENT

PROBLEM: HIGH FOREHEAD, BORING COLOR

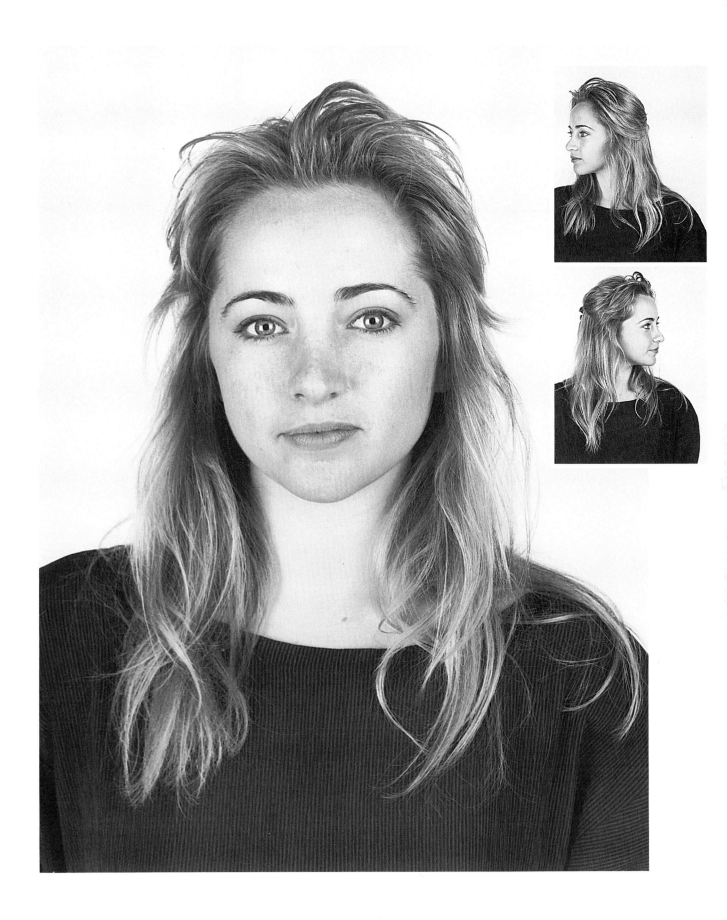

I think Tara is typical of many women. There really wasn't anything wrong with her at all. She was young, pretty, and bright. But she didn't look as good as she could have. She wasn't maximizing her potential. When you maximize your potential, whatever that potential is, people will notice you. For Tara, who was studying to become an actress, being noticed was very important. Tara did not have to be drop-dead gorgeous in order to be a successful actress. As we discussed earlier, the really good actresses of today aren't gorgeous at all. (Fortunately, the theater-going public seems to require more than just a pretty face to be entertained these days.) But Tara *did* need to be interesting-looking. She had to possess that certain sparkle that attracts people's attention right away.

When I asked Tara what she was looking for from a makeover, she said exactly what I wanted to hear: "I want to look unique."

I knew I could help Tara get what she wanted—after all, she was already very attractive. I just wanted her to have her own look, her own sense of style—not a poor imitation of someone else's. . . .

I liked Tara's blond hair, but I didn't love it. The problem was that the color had become sort of dishwater, very nondescript. This would never do. If there is one thing I can't stand, it is hair that looks ordinary. If Tara was to stay a blonde, she had to be an exciting blonde! I thus decided to give her brighter, lighter highlights using a combination of bleach and golden coloring, highlights that would accent the blue of her eyes.

After seeing the smile on Tara's face when we finished, I knew we had made the right decision about hair-coloring. But the thing to remember about Tara—and this is true for every woman I work with—is that we did what we did for her the day she came in because it was the right thing for her *at that time.* If Tara were to come back to me next year, we very well might not do the same thing. Maybe I'd make her a redhead or a brunette. This is not an exact science. Sometimes it's simply a matter of just feeling or sensing what you need to look beautiful *at that moment.*

Tara very much wanted to keep her hair long. Like many women, she enjoyed being able to wear her hair in many different styles to accommodate her different moods. There's nothing wrong with that. But in Tara's case whatever style we chose had to be fun and carefree and spirited. After all, what better time of life is there to look alive and playful than when you are twenty or twenty-one? It's only at that age that you have the opportunity to look both innocent and sexy at the same time. I wanted to capture that in Tara.

Tara had a great jawline, distinct but not too angular. She also had nice high cheekbones. In order to draw attention to these assets, I cut her hair blunt at the sides and fringed the ends (that is, cut them in jagged layers) all around her face. The idea was to shape her hair so that it would silhouette the shape of her face. The eye is naturally drawn to the place where the hair ends and the skin begins.

Tara wanted to grow out her bangs, but I dissuaded her from that. Because she had such a high forehead (at least in comparison to the rest of her head), she needed bangs to create the illusion that her head was perfectly proportioned.

The result was striking. What had been a pretty but rather ordinary young girl was now a striking child/woman who could easily capture the attention of anyone she chose.

What's more, Tara won't be late for any auditions—at least not because of her new hairdo. It is as easy to maintain as it is attractive.

DOING IT YOURSELF

TOOLS NEEDED: Mousse, vent brush, large-size rough brush, blow dryer, hair spray.

To maintain this look, you begin by applying a small amount of mousse to clean, wet hair. Then you tip your head down and blow-dry your hair, brushing it continuously with the vent brush. When it is only slightly damp, straighten up and finish blow-drying it, using the large round brush to bend the ends slightly toward your face. Finally, mess your hair with your hands and allow it to fall back into place naturally, then hold the style with hair spray.

If you want, you can give yourself a really curly look by using a medium-size curling iron or medium-size hot rollers all over your head.

TARA'S COMMENTS

I love my new look, I really do. I was sure that Jose would want to cut my hair off and that if I asked him not to, he'd say forget it. But he understood completely and made my hair look better than it ever had before. I really do feel like I have my own identity, that I'm not stuck looking like everyone else.

The one thing I've noticed the most about people is that they seem to be awfully fickle. When I go out feeling like I look great, people treat me fantastic. If I go out the very next night and run into the very same people, *not* looking so great, believe me, they don't treat me fantastic.

It seems that some people only want to be seen with good-looking men and women around them. It's very humbling when you think you've made a new friend one minute and the next minute your new *friend* won't give you the time of day. What does it take to convince people to go deeper, to learn more and try harder? The riches received from an internal relationship are far more precious than the temporary riches people think they receive from a *physical* relationship.

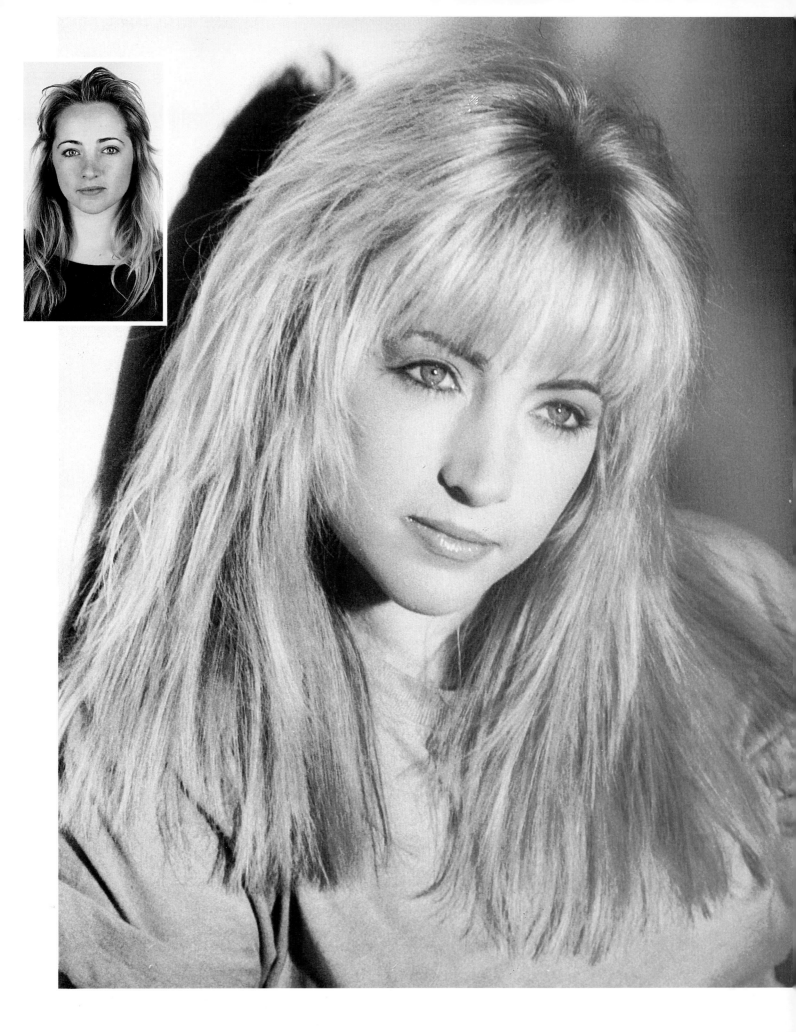

3

FROM VALLEY GIRL TO UPTOWN GIRL

R I A
H A N D E L S

AGE: 21

OCCUPATION:

WAITRESS

PROBLEM:

STRINGY, LIFELESS,

ORDINARY-

LOOKING HAIR

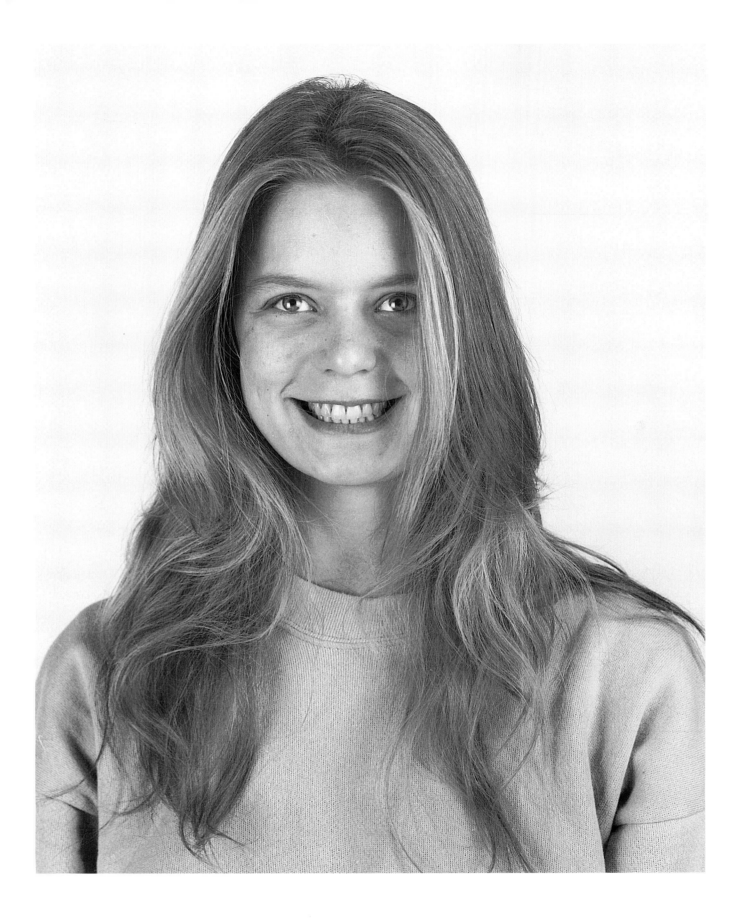

When I met Ria for the first time, I saw the potential for a major beauty. I knew she had no idea how pretty she was, and I was very excited about showing her. When I asked Ria what she did for a living, she told me she worked as a waitress. I noticed her accent and discovered she had recently moved back to California after living most of her life in Brussels. Upon further investigation I learned that Ria had come to Los Angeles all by herself in hopes of becoming a model. Although Ria is a native Californian, it was so long since she'd left Los Angeles that she was really alone here, without family or friends. I understood what she was going through, and I admired her strength of character.

Ria's only problem was that she had allowed herself to look ordinary. She admitted to wearing her hair long and straight every day. For work, she would tie it back in a ponytail to keep it away from the food she was serving, but that was the only variation—ever. I teased Ria, calling her our Valley girl. I promised her that if she would just *trust* me, I would change her from a Valley girl to an uptown girl. She did. . . .

Why is it that women always think hairstylists automatically want to cut off their hair? It seems as if every woman with medium-length hair and beyond who sits in my chair invariably asks, "You're not going to cut it short, are you?" As if I were going to strap them down, gag their mouths, and scalp them. In case you haven't noticed, I love long hair! Well, let's say

I love long hair when it is clean, conditioned, and coiffed. Believe me, when a woman can wear long hair, I encourage it.

Ria was one of those women. The only thing I did to the length of her hair was trim the ends in order to get rid of some damage. Otherwise, I left it long.

What Ria's hair really needed, far more than trimming, was volume, body, and pizzazz. And the fastest, easiest way to achieve that is with a perm. There are several different types of perms to choose from, depending on the amount of wave you want and the type of hair you have. I felt Ria should have very soft, loose, ringlets that would make her look more sophisticated without diminishing her youth and spirit. So I suggested a spiral perm. A spiral perm is rolled vertically with thick, rubber rods in an unconstructed manner. The result is a natural, free-flowing, feminine-looking wave.

I really liked the natural, sun-touched color of Ria's hair. Sometimes Mother Nature takes care of us and we don't have to add any additional color at all. Another time we might like to see Ria as a brunette, but for now her hair color suited her just fine. Of course, the chemical process of a permanent wave lightens hair automatically; there is no way to avoid that. Fortunately, the effect is not dramatic; certainly, it didn't change Ria's color too drastically.

Though the change in Ria was quite remarkable, the process was really quite simple. All we really did was give her a perm. I don't know of any style that is easier to take care of than Ria's. Her hair can look fabulous without any effort on her part.

DOING IT YOURSELF

TOOLS NEEDED: Mousse, comb or pick, blow dryer, diffuser, hair spray.

After shampooing this perm, you go through your hair with a comb or pick simply to untangle it. For a little extra body, add a touch of mousse to your roots. That's it. You don't have to do anything else. You can let your hair dry naturally and style it with your fingers. If you don't want to leave the house with a wet head, you can blow-dry your hair using a diffuser to keep it from frizzing. A little finger styling, a squirt of hair spray, and you're finished. Fast and easy.

I can't stress enough the extent to which small changes can make a big difference. All we did was perm Ria's hair, and she looked entirely different. She had energy and life and interest. She looked confident and eager to take on the world. When Ria walked into my salon she had dreams of *becoming* a model. When she walked out of my salon she felt she *was* a model.

RIA'S COMMENTS

I was probably the only person in Los Angeles who didn't know of Jose Eber. The truth is I had never heard of the man before. Having lived in Brussels, I wasn't familiar with him or his work. But I knew if I was ever going to get a modeling job, I had to make myself look more interesting. One of the few friends I'd made since moving to Los Angeles told me of Jose's reputation, that he was the best hairdresser anywhere. I had absolutely nothing to lose, so I decided to give it a try.

My friend told me Jose was good but said nothing to me about his appearance. I was fascinated by this man with a cowboy hat and a long braid who captivated all the women who showed up for makeovers. After talking to me for a little while, Jose said I looked like a Valley girl. I could tell he was teasing me, but I had no idea what a Valley girl was. Then he told me he could make me look beautiful, and I could tell he wasn't teasing at all. I was grateful for the attention. I was grateful that someone seemed to care about me in Los Angeles. I told Jose that I wanted to be a model. He didn't laugh. Instead, he made me look like one.

There are many things we can do to improve our outer beauty. We can exercise, wear makeup, buy a new outfit, or change our hairstyle. All of these things do wonders for the exterior. I wish there were a checklist as simple for improving the interior.

People seem to be satisfied with their first impressions. If they don't like the way someone looks, most of the time they don't even bother to find out what that person has to offer on the inside. To me, this is very sad. That may sound funny coming from a person who wants to be a model, but that's the way I feel. If things go well for me, modeling will be my career. But liking people for the way they look only works in front of the camera. I wouldn't dream of basing a friendship on physical appearance, at least not anymore. Like most people, I made the mistake of doing that in the past and was really hurt. I honestly believe that's one lesson you have to experience in order to learn. Too bad, because it's very painful.

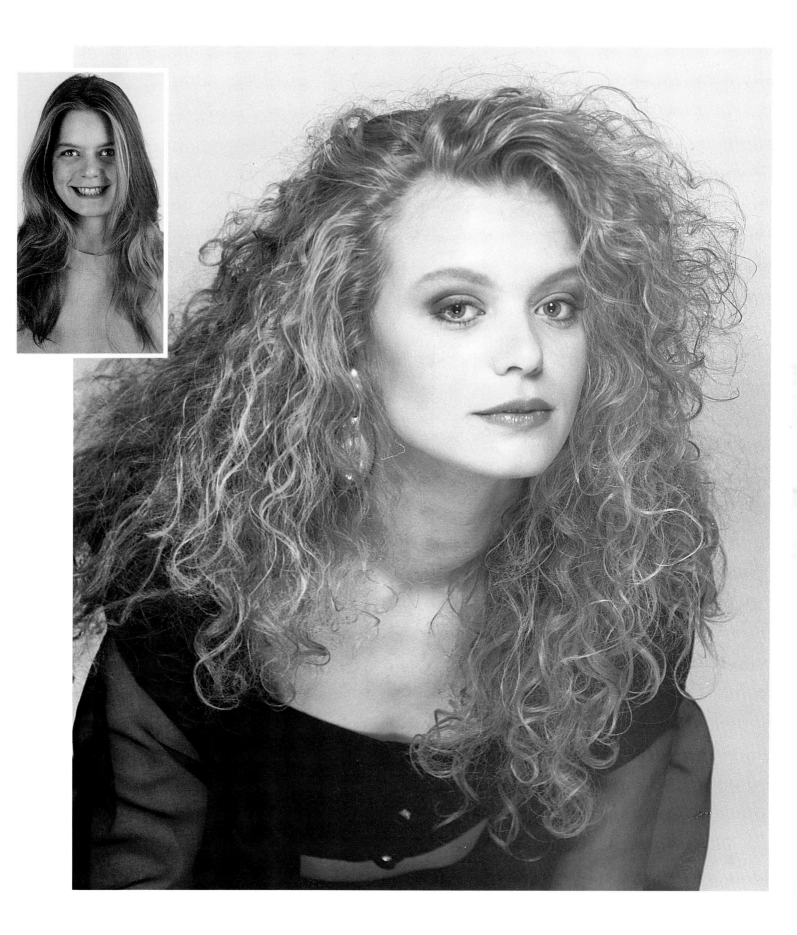

4

TAKING A SHORT CUT

DEBBIE SRIBERG

AGE: 27

OCCUPATION:
PSYCHOLOGICAL
COUNSELOR

PROBLEM:
LONG FACE,
CLOSE-SET EYES

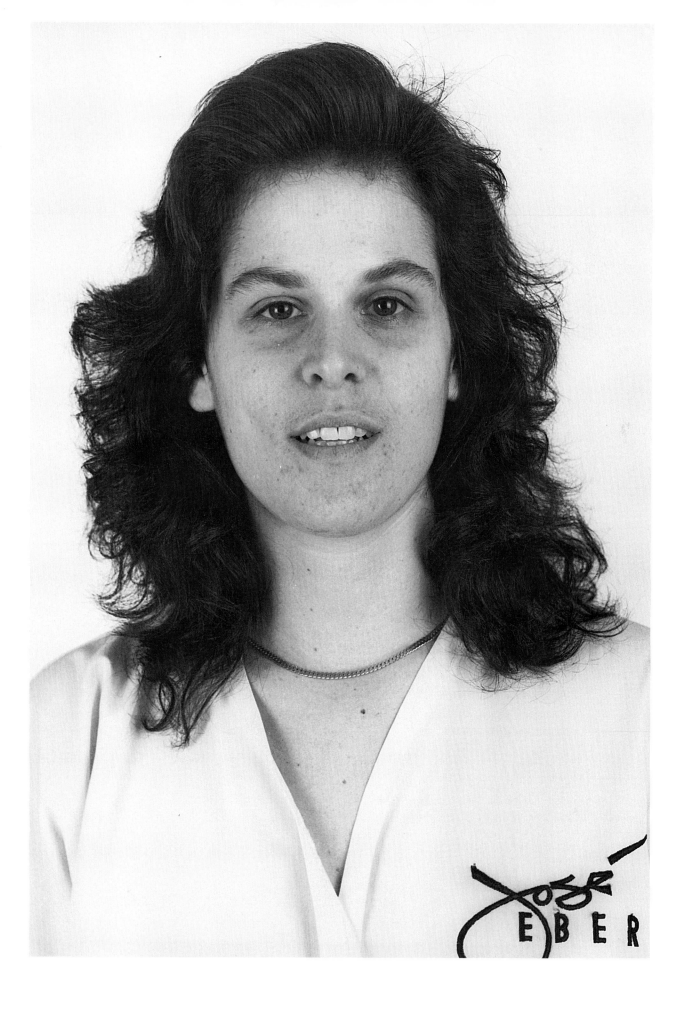

D E B B I E   S R I B E R G

On the night of the open call when I chose the women who appear in this book, Debbie was the first one in the door. She was also the first one to be chosen. I remember being somewhat surprised that she had come. I really don't know why; she just didn't seem the type to go in for a make-over. But I do know that I liked her right away. Debbie had a hint of mischief in her eyes and mannerisms that I found quite amusing. I knew that I could make her look a lot more polished without much difficulty. My concern was finding a sufficiently easy look for Debbie; I didn't want it to be so much trouble to maintain that she wouldn't bother to keep it up afterward.

Debbie told me that she had two jobs. By day she assisted college students in need of psychological counseling, and by night she worked as a community-service counselor in a residential treatment program. That meant that whatever style I gave her had to be fast and had to be easy. Debbie wasn't the type to fuss in front of the mirror all morning. Still, she wanted to look better.

Just like Ria, the first thing Debbie asked me when she sat down on my chair was, "You're not going to cut it short, are you?" I told her that, of course, I wouldn't cut it short if she didn't want me to. Actually, short hair can be a lot more work than long hair. You can always tie long hair back when you don't want to fuss with it. For that reason alone, given Debbie's busy schedule, I would have probably opted for a longer style. But just as we were deciding, my friend Ali MacGraw walked in the salon and sat down on the chair right next to Debbie. Debbie and I both looked at Ali and knew that hers was the cut we wanted. The look was short, smart, and not too delicate. The perfect thing for Debbie.

Before we cut Debbie's hair, I made a slight adjustment to its color. Her combination of olive skin and dark hair gave her a tendency to look a little harsh. To soften her look a bit, I touched up her hair with a hint of copper highlights. This did not change the color, it just made her hair a little warmer and a little shinier. I used a nonperoxide type of coloring so that if Debbie didn't make it back to the salon for a while, she wouldn't be bothered with dark roots. Nonperoxide color fades away gradually with each washing.

Ali MacGraw's short hairstyle was just right for Debbie for a number of reasons. To begin with, Debbie has a long face, and a cut like Ali's that features heavy bangs on the forehead is an ideal way to make a long face look shorter. Bangs are also good for camouflaging eyes that, like Debbie's, are a bit close-set. The secret is to make the bangs long enough to cover the eyebrows. Finally, Debbie has great cheekbones—and a style like Ali's, in which the hair is cut away from the face, draws the eye outward toward them.

This style may not be as easy to maintain as a longer cut, which you can just throw back into a ponytail. But it can still look great in no time at all.

DOING IT YOURSELF

TOOLS NEEDED: Mousse, vent brush, blow dryer, hair spray.

After applying a little mousse to the roots of your clean, wet hair, all you have to do to maintain this style is bend your head over and blow-dry your hair with a vent brush. That's it. No round brush, curling iron, or hot roller.

Debbie's makeover created a lot of excitement in the salon. Nobody could get over the dramatic change. Even Ali was excited!

DEBBIE'S COMMENTS

I had never had a makeover in my life, never really wanted one. But for some reason I had been contemplating a change in my appearance. When Jose agreed to do me, I was so excited and nervous. What had I gotten myself into?

I have never understood why so much emphasis is placed on the way people look. I mean why it is more important than the way people are. I guess I've noticed it more since moving to Los Angeles, but it's the same everywhere. People get so hung up on physical beauty, but physical beauty isn't what makes you laugh or cry or think. That requires inner beauty.

We all like to look at attractive people, and we all like to be thought of as attractive. Thanks to Jose, I feel attractive for the first time in my life. But I am twenty-seven years old. It would be pretty sad if I had had to wait until I thought I looked good in order to be happy. My whole life up until now would have been a waste. Fortunately, I relied on my inner self for happiness. That's also what I looked for in others. To me, beauty is being yourself and allowing others to be themselves—without judgment. Of course, there's no harm in being the best self you can be—on the inside *and* the outside. I know now that's what brought me to Jose's salon.

I could never conform to the California image—even if I wanted to. I'm not thin, blond, and bikinis. I'm big, brown, and boxer shorts. And that's the way I like it.

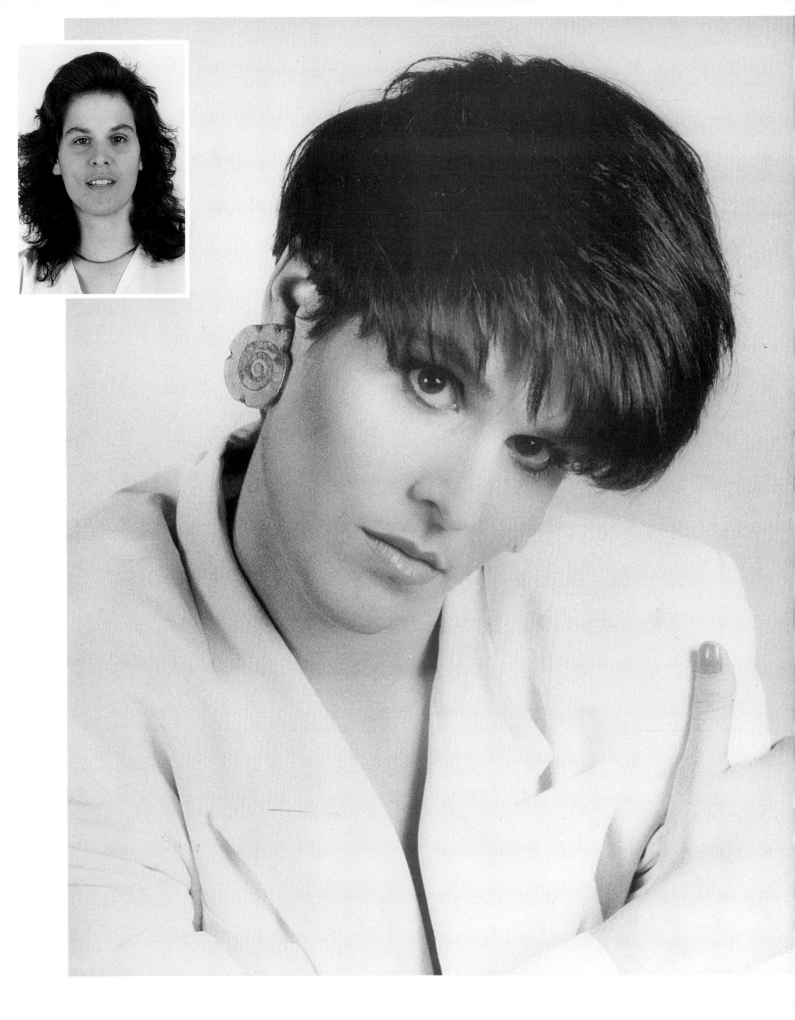

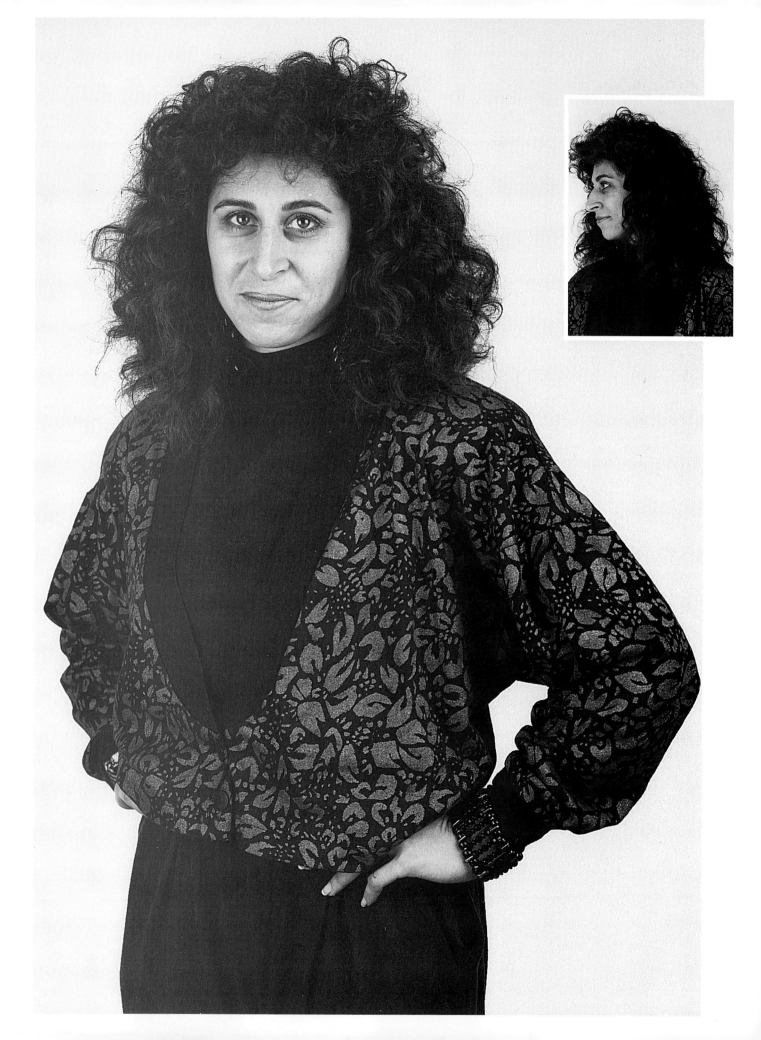

5

COMING OUT OF HIDING

ROSINE HATEM

AGE: 29

OCCUPATION:

WAITRESS/ STUNTWOMAN

PROBLEM:

LONG NOSE,

WILD CURLY HAIR

I first noticed Rosine walk in my salon out of the corner of my eye. It took me a while to get over to her, but I kept thinking, This woman has such an interesting look, I must speak to her. When I got closer to Rosine and saw that fabulous nose and that million-dollar smile, I knew I had to make her face more easily accessible to the world. It was completely buried under her bushy hair.

I have always been fascinated by faces with a lot of character, faces with unique, captivating features. To me, Rosine had a nose to be shown off. To me, her nose was beautiful. But not to Rosine. I had the impression that consciously or subconsciously she was hiding her nose behind big masses of curly hair. Of course, whenever people think you're trying to hide something, they become much more curious and much more interested in what that something might be. It's human nature.

Rosine has the sort of personality that attracts people. She is fun, adventurous, and sensitive. As a waitress, she is in constant contact with the public. And as a stuntwoman, she must exude a sense of ease and confidence. Given all that, I thought it was a shame that she wasn't more confident about her appearance.

I couldn't wait to get started on Rosine because I knew just how good she would look when I was done. The first thing that had to go was that curly mop of hair behind which she hid her face. Specifically, I thinned her hair at the sides and in the back. I did leave a lot of volume on top, but I shortened the length. The immediate effect of this was to redirect attention away from her hair and onto her face, where it belonged. It also exposed Rosine's gorgeous neck. Her neck, which is long and graceful, deserved to be shown off. Before the cut, it had gone completely unnoticed. Finally, giving her hair a little height on the top made Rosine look taller and slimmer.

But the most dramatic change in Rosine's appearance came when we altered her hair color. With her small frame and strong features, her dark hair looked too harsh. I suggested a lighter shade, a light mahogany, to complement her olive skin. It looked wonderful.

Rosine came out looking like a woman in command. Instead of appearing wild and unkempt, she seemed pulled together and organized. Her hair was no longer in control—she was. What's more, her exquisite jawline and cheekbones and her lovely complexion—none of which I'll bet you noticed in the "before" picture—finally were getting the attention they deserved.

As I mentioned before, when I style someone's hair, I always leave the ultimate decision on what should be done up to the client. Of course, I make suggestions, and I generally have good reasons for them. But I would never insist that someone let me do something to her hair that makes her feel uncomfortable. Nor would I ever "surprise" a client with an unexpected new look.

The reason for this is simple. In order for a style to be really effective, it not only must look sensational, it also must make the client happy. That means it must fit in with her life-style and jibe with her self-image.

Still, every once in a while, despite all the consultations, the initial shock of a new style can be quite overwhelming for a client. That was the case with Rosine. When she first saw how much shorter her hair was, she panicked a bit. There were even a few tears. I understood how she felt. I hugged her and suggested that she look in the mirror and give herself a chance to become acquainted with that fabulous face she had been previously trying to hide.

Before very long, Rosine seemed to take on a new air of confidence and self-acceptance. Then the tears were for a different reason.

The truth is, Rosine was always an interesting-looking woman. But now she looks and acts as if she's proud of her appearance.

What's more, her new style requires almost no maintenance at all—an important consideration for someone as active and busy as Rosine.

DOING IT YOURSELF

TOOLS NEEDED: Gel, blow dryer with diffuser (optional), hair spray.

To maintain this style, you begin by applying some gel—from the roots to the tips—while your hair is still wet. This adds a little weight to the curls, keeping them under control. We let Rosine's hair dry naturally, but if you are in a hurry, you can use a blow dryer. Just be sure to attach a diffuser. This will keep your curls from becoming too wild. When your hair is completely dry, use your fingers to fluff up the top. A touch of hair spray and you're done. What could be easier?

ROSINE'S COMMENTS

When I heard Jose was looking for people to give makeovers to, I thought, Great—this is just the guy I've always wanted to do my hair. When we finally met, I was surprised at his candor. He talked about my long nose and bushy hair in the same breath as he said I was beautiful. He made me feel good. Even when I got upset, he remained calm and confident. Yet he was so sensitive to my feelings. He didn't make me feel silly or foolish for crying. He stood there and hugged me, and then he introduced me to this really pretty woman I'd never met before—Rosine Hatem.

Inner beauty is the only thing that can really make people happy. It is the ability to make intimate contact with another person. Not physically intimate, but spiritually intimate. To leave a person feeling better for having met you.

I think to have inner beauty you have to have self-esteem. You have to be confident about the things you do and pleased with the way you treat other people. I think Jose has inner beauty, but more important he *gives* people inner beauty. That might sound funny since he is famous for giving people outer beauty. But that's what makes him different from other hairdressers. He knows that a woman will never look good on the outside if she doesn't feel good on the inside, so he works on the soul at the same time he works on the hair. And you never see it coming.

There are a lot of ugly people out there who fool you constantly because they look pretty good. And then there are a lot of really beautiful people out there to whom you'd never give the time of day because they don't look so good. When this happens, who's the fool?

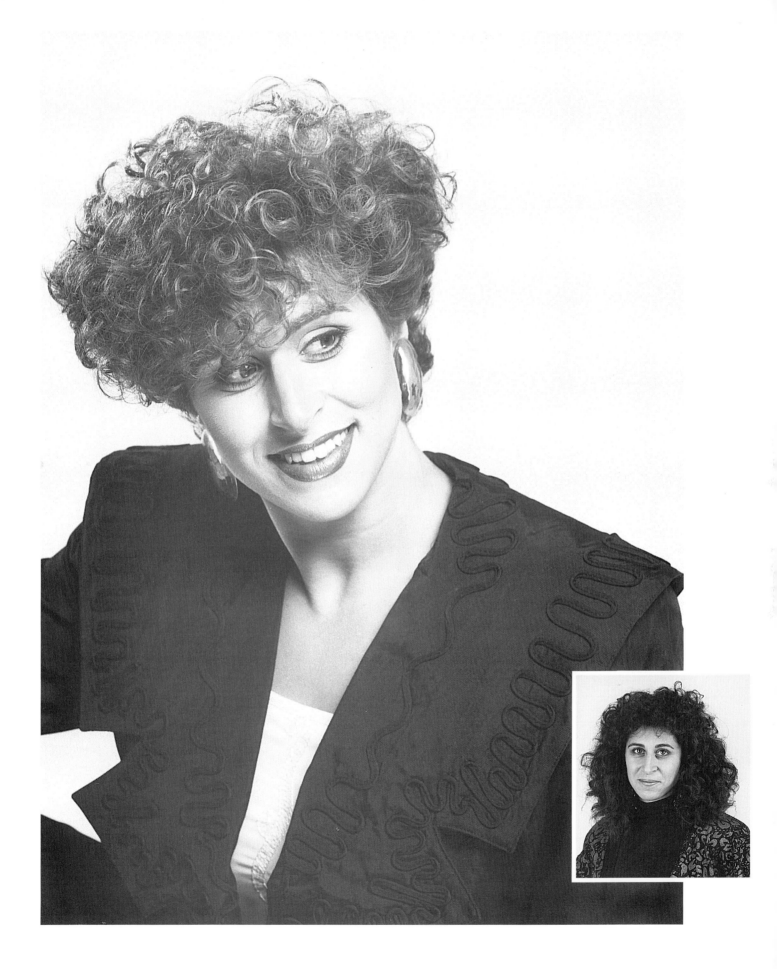

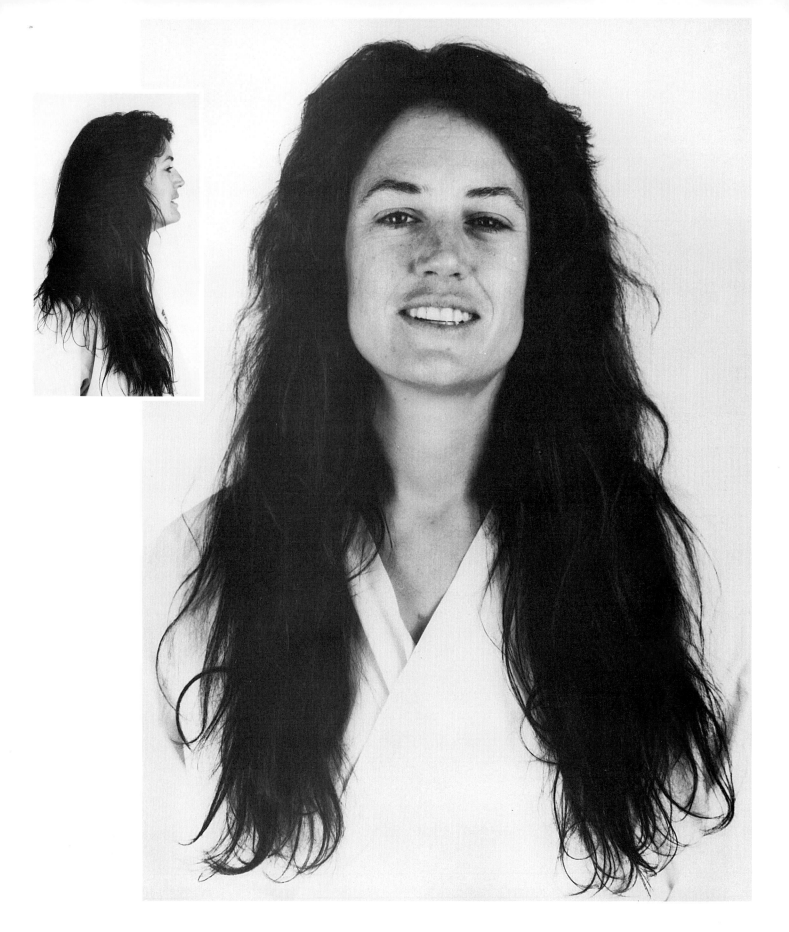

6

TOO MUCH OF A GOOD THING

DIANE GRANT McGROARTY

AGE: 31

OCCUPATION:
STUNTWOMAN

PROBLEM:
LONG FACE,
NARROW FOREHEAD

DIANE GRANT McGROARTY

When a woman who stands six feet two inches tall walks into my salon, you can bet I'm going to notice her. And when she tells me she's a stuntwoman, you can bet my interest is going to be piqued. When I first saw Diane, I just kept looking up—until I got to her face. I loved her look.

When I asked Diane why she had come to see me, what she wanted to change about the way she looked, she said she honestly didn't know. I have found that to be true of many of the women who come to see me. Diane felt she could look better than she did, but she didn't know exactly what needed to be done to make that happen.

In talking to her a little more about her life-style, I learned that Diane leads a very active life—more active than most. She is a stuntwoman, a wife (married to a stuntman), and the mother of a three-year-old daughter. A typical day for her might include a car explosion, a plane crash, a shoot-out, and a nursery rhyme (not necessarily in that order). It would be a challenge for me to find a hairstyle that could keep up with her. But I knew there was a soft side to this woman, and I wanted to bring it out. . . .

o o o

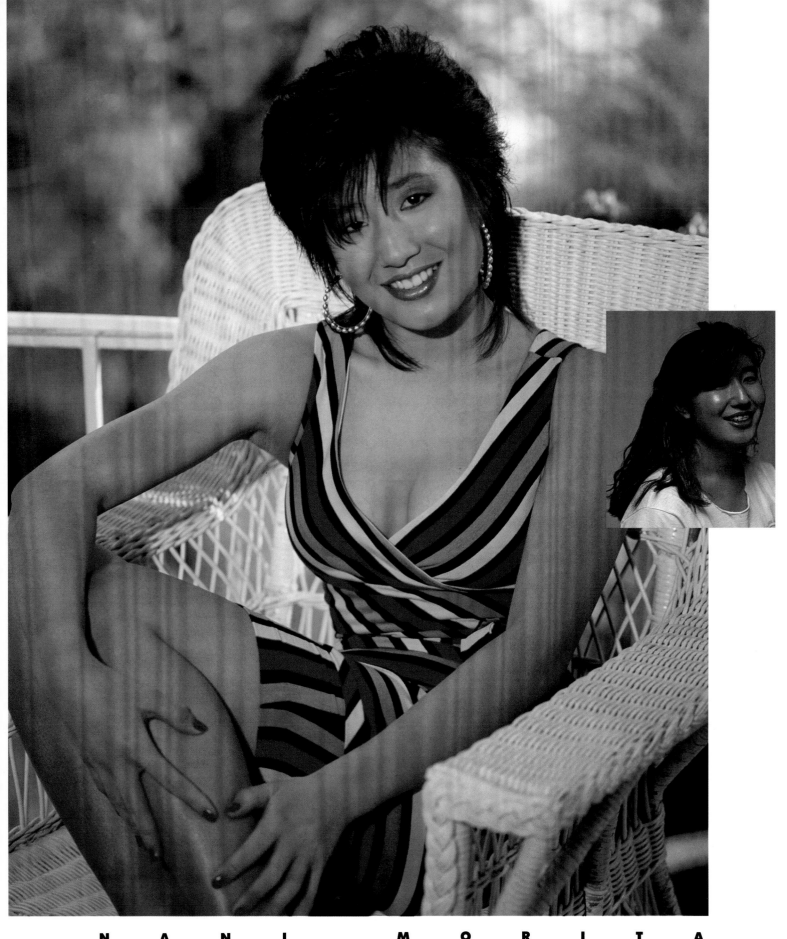

N A N I   M O R I T A

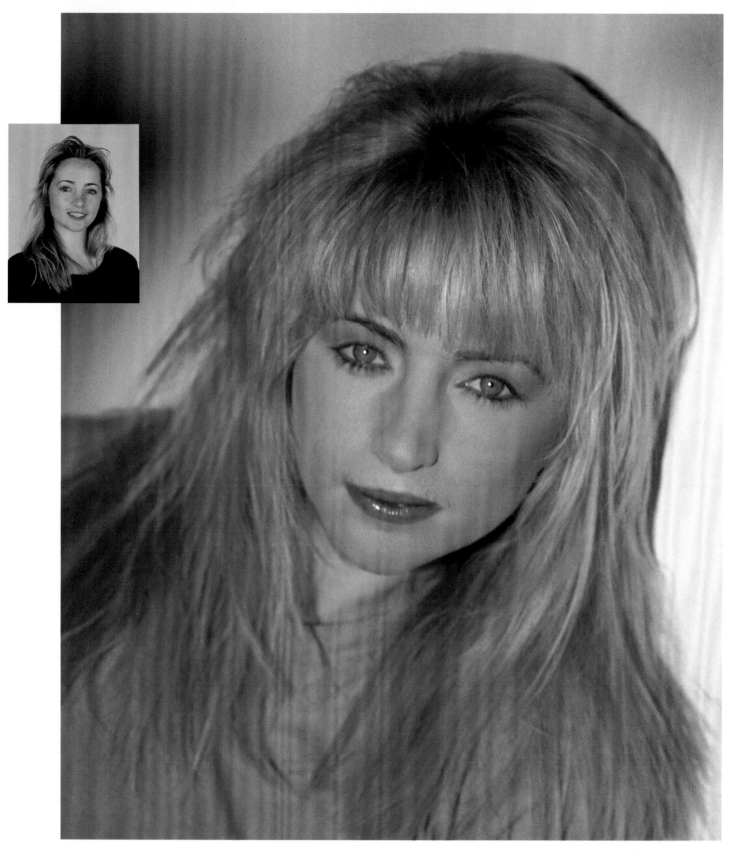

T A R A   E L L I S O N

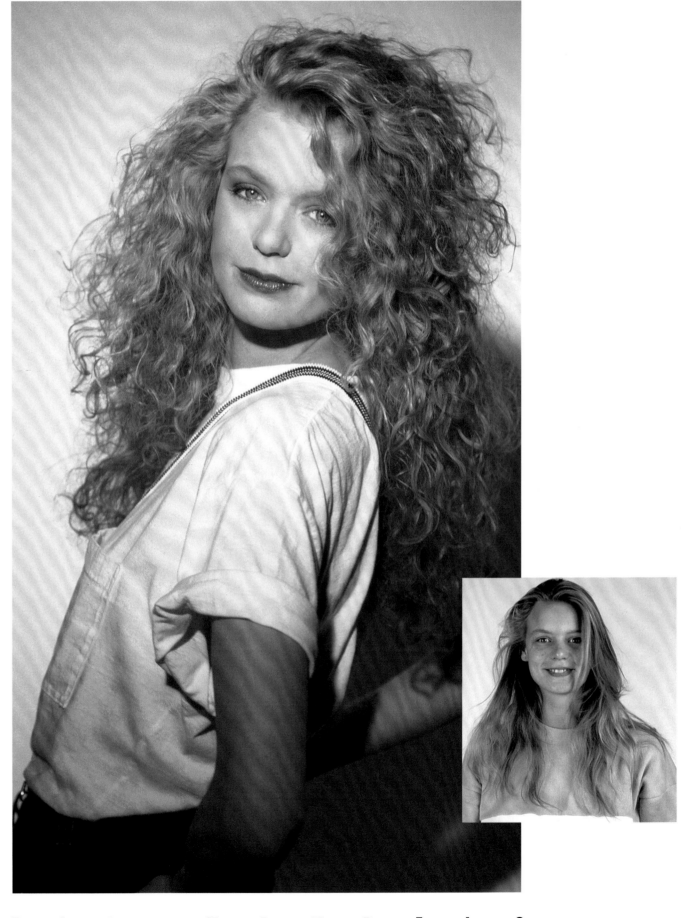

R I A   H A N D E L S

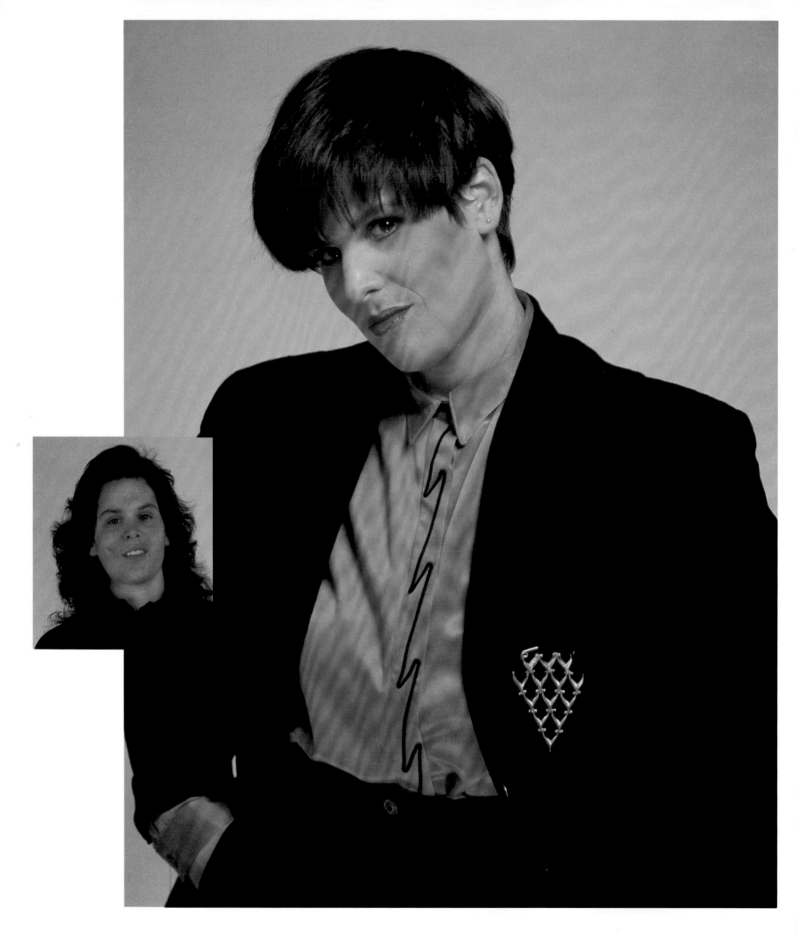

D E B B I E   S R I B E R G

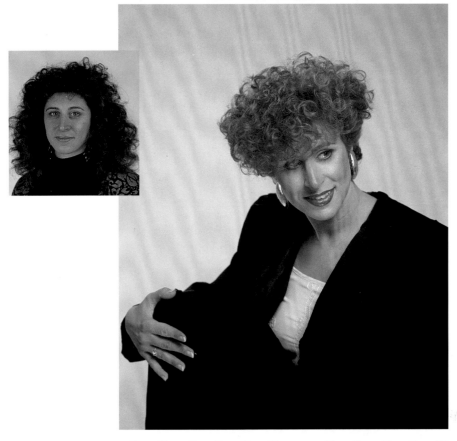

ROSINE HATEM

DIANE GRANT McGROARTY

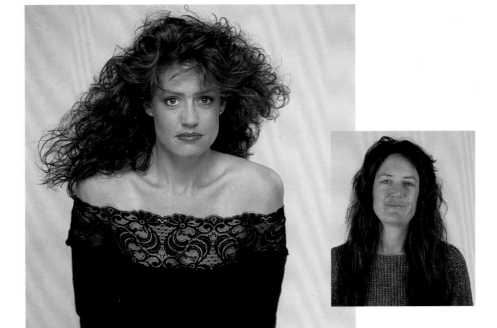

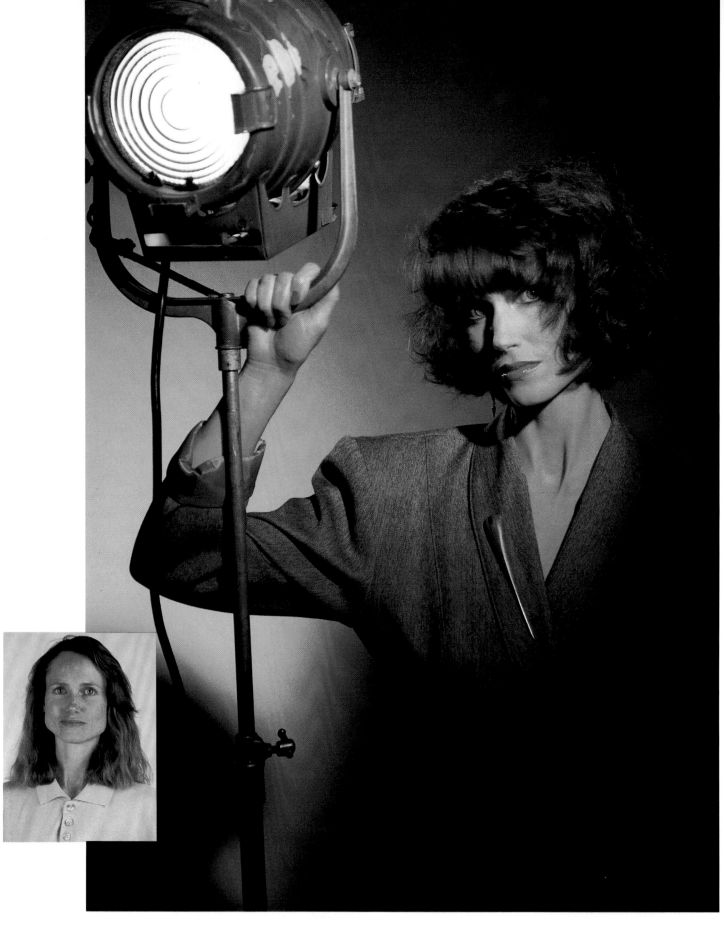

M O L L I E   R A T O

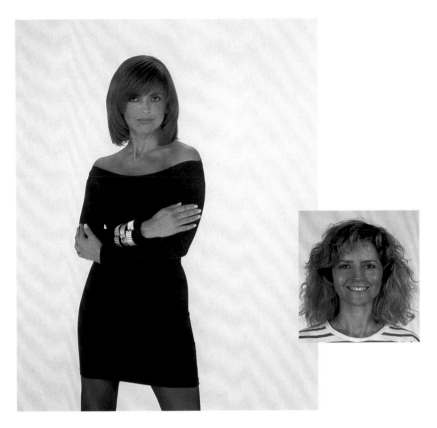

D E B B I E   H E N R Y

P A M   S H A W

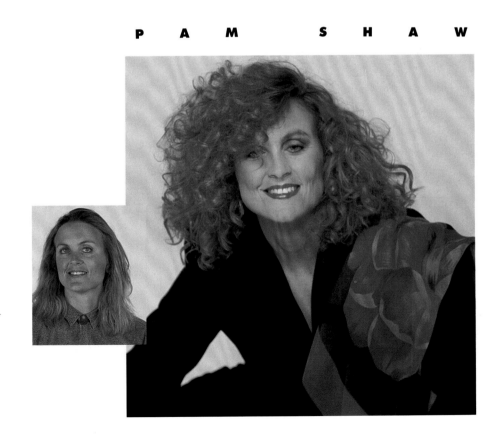

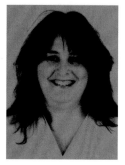

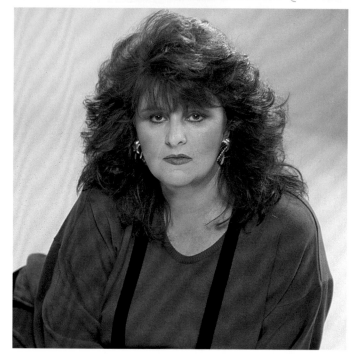

CATHERINE KENNEDY

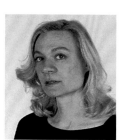

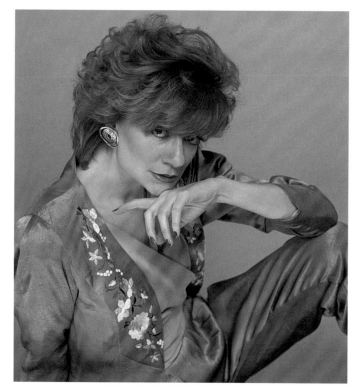

SANDRA MILLER

FAYE BELAND

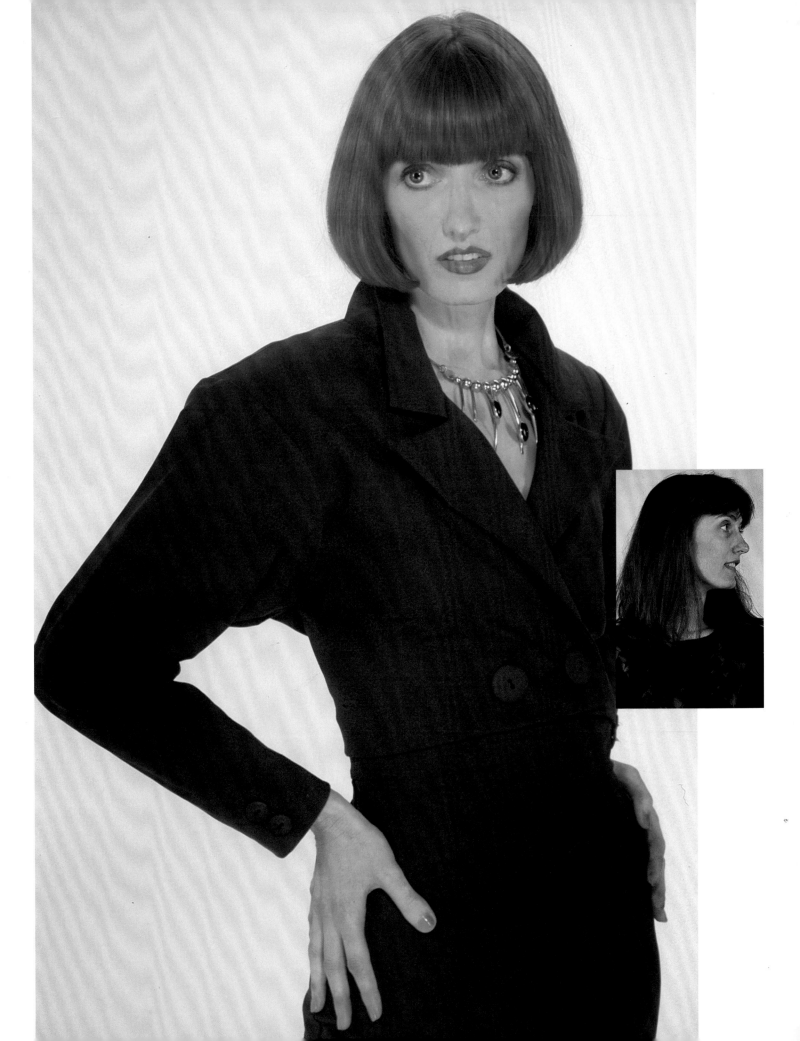

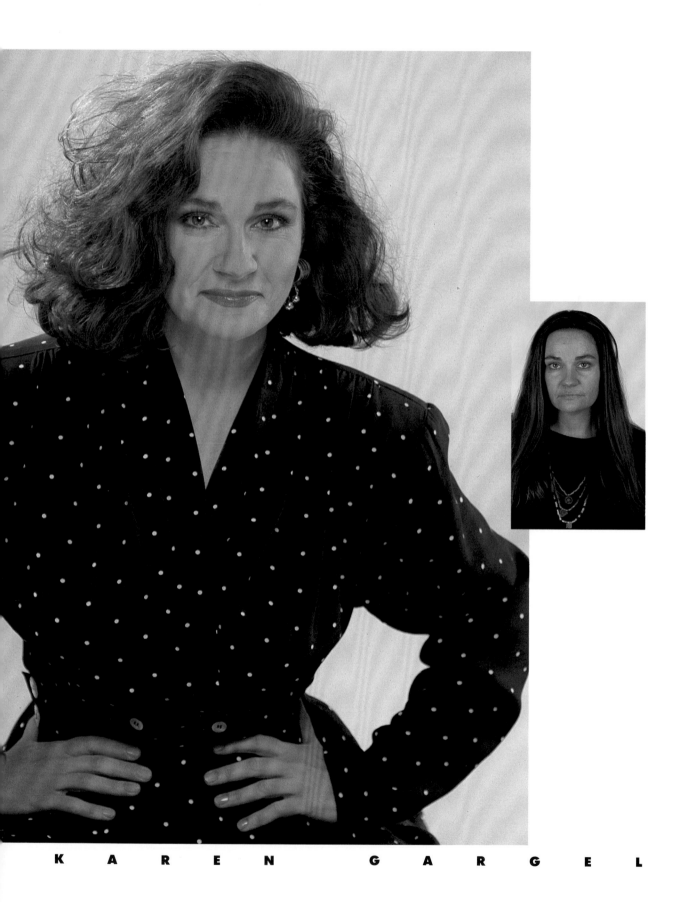

K A R E N G A R G E L

JOHNETTA BUSH

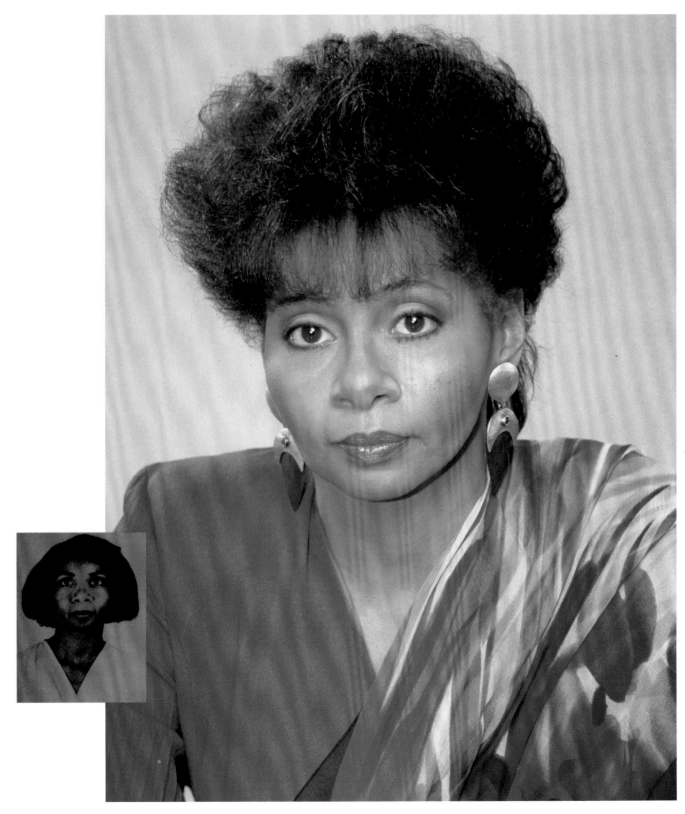

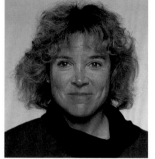

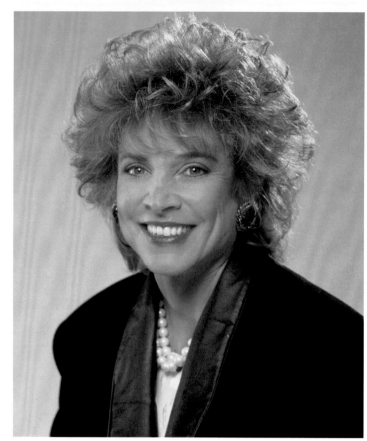

D A N A   H E N R Y

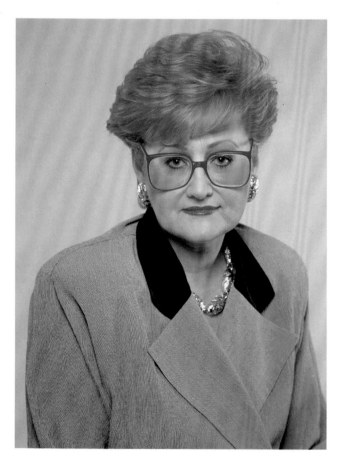

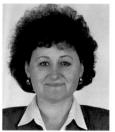

C. G.   O'C O N N O R

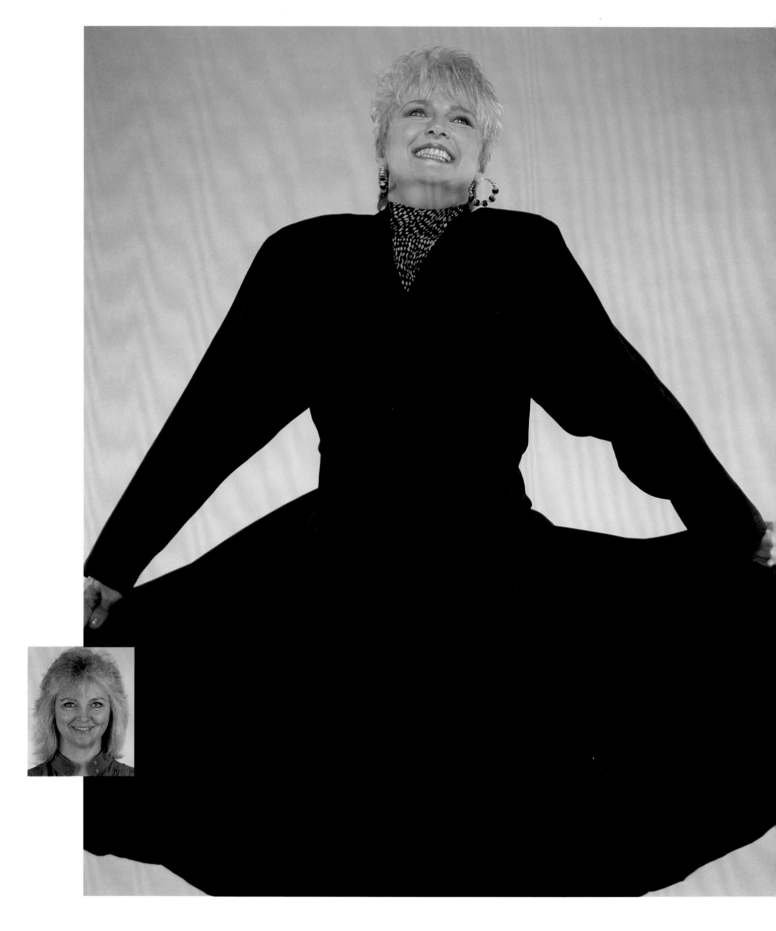

D'ANN FRASCA SNYDER

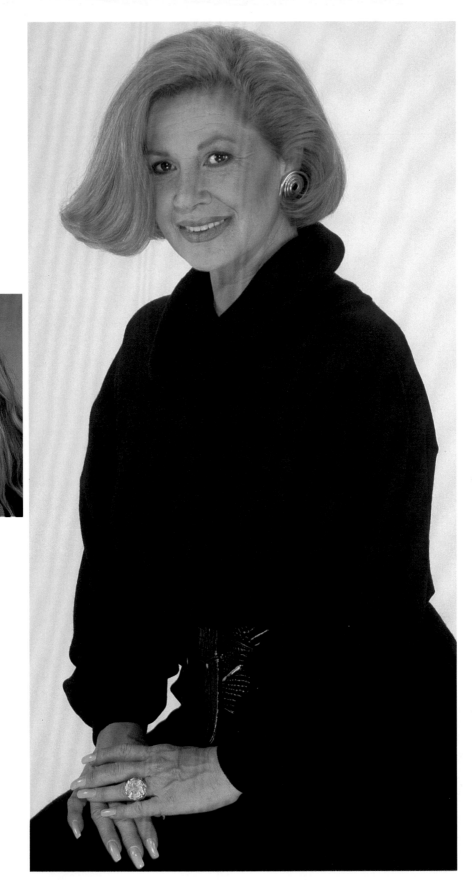

L O R R A I N E   P E T T I T

S A L L Y   F A R V E R

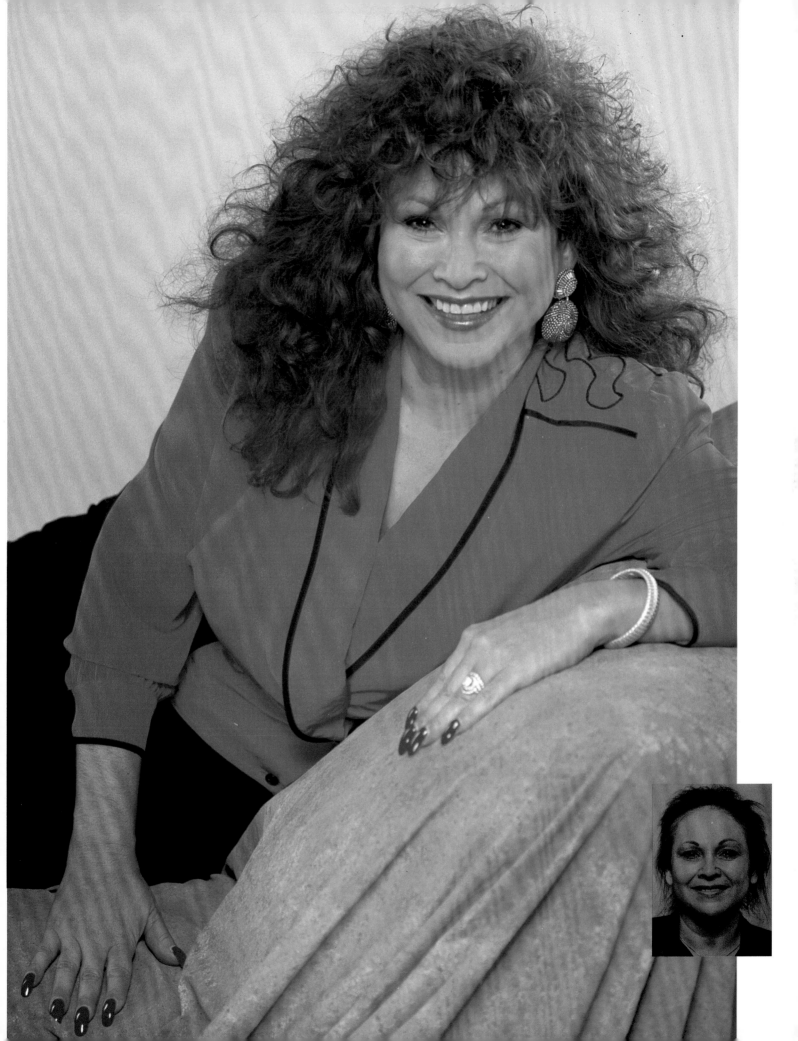

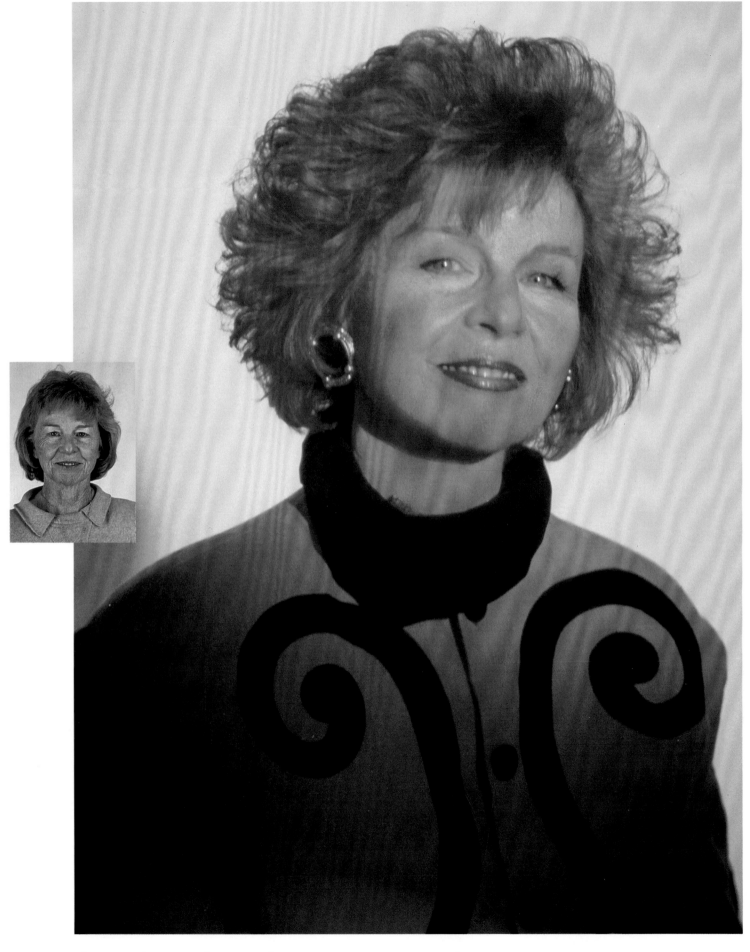

C A R O   J O N E S

Obviously, the first thing anyone notices about Diane is her height. The problem with her old look was that her hair hung just like her body—long and straight. It wasn't the most flattering style for Diane, nor was it the most feminine.

Though you would have never known it, Diane has naturally wavy hair. Unfortunately she wore it so long that its weight flattened out its natural body. So the first thing I did was to shorten it by four or five inches. (I would have taken off a bit more, but Diane wanted to leave it long enough so she could put it in a braid; apparently the many wigs she uses in her job stay anchored better when they're put on over a braid.) Taking off those four or five inches allowed her hair to bounce back immediately. To bring fullness to the sides, I did a lot of layering.

Diane looked gorgeous as a brunette, so I didn't suggest any major changes in her color. Still, I felt that lightening her hair a couple of shades would make her look a little softer, a little more gentle. It did, bringing out the feminine side of Diane—the mother, the wife. She may have walked into my salon a stuntwoman, but she walked out a very sexy lady. The best thing about her new look is that it is practically wash-and-wear.

DOING IT YOURSELF

TOOLS NEEDED: Mousse, comb, blow dryer, hair spray.

The first thing you do after shampooing is add a little mousse to your roots for extra body. Then comb through your hair quickly just to get out the tangles. While blow-drying, grab small sections of your hair and scrunch them up in little balls, holding them in place until they are completely dry. This is an easy way to liven up naturally wavy hair without bothering with hot rollers or a curling iron. As far as the bangs are concerned, just pull them forward and allow them to dry straight. A touch of hair spray for safekeeping, and, like Diane, you're ready for God only knows what.

I think the "new" Diane looks beautiful. Of course, I thought she was pretty impressive to start with.

DIANE'S COMMENTS

My last experience in a salon was a total disaster. I allowed someone to give me a perm that turned out so badly I ended up crying all the way home. I cried so hard that I couldn't see where I was going and got a traffic ticket in the process. The funny thing was that Jose showed me that my hair doesn't even *need* a perm.

When you are as active and crazy as I am, you don't often take the time to stop and think about looking pretty. Even if I did have the time, up until I met Jose I wouldn't have known how. He was the first one to actually *teach* me how to make myself look my best. I still may not do it every day, but I have the knowledge and the ability to capture that same look any time I want to.

It's a good feeling to know how to be pretty.

In my opinion, far too much emphasis is placed on a woman's size. I'm lucky because I'm tall enough to carry weight without looking fat. But I know people who starve themselves just to stay thin—to the point where their lives are in jeopardy. They are convinced that if they were to become fat, they would be social outcasts and be less loved. The sad thing is that may be true. I will never understand why people judge other people in that way.

I think inner beauty comes from feeling good about the way you communicate with other people. And just as you can work on your outer beauty by fixing your hair, wearing makeup, or dressing up, you can also work on your inner beauty by taking an active interest in other people, by giving of yourself when your help is needed, and by setting a good example for young children.

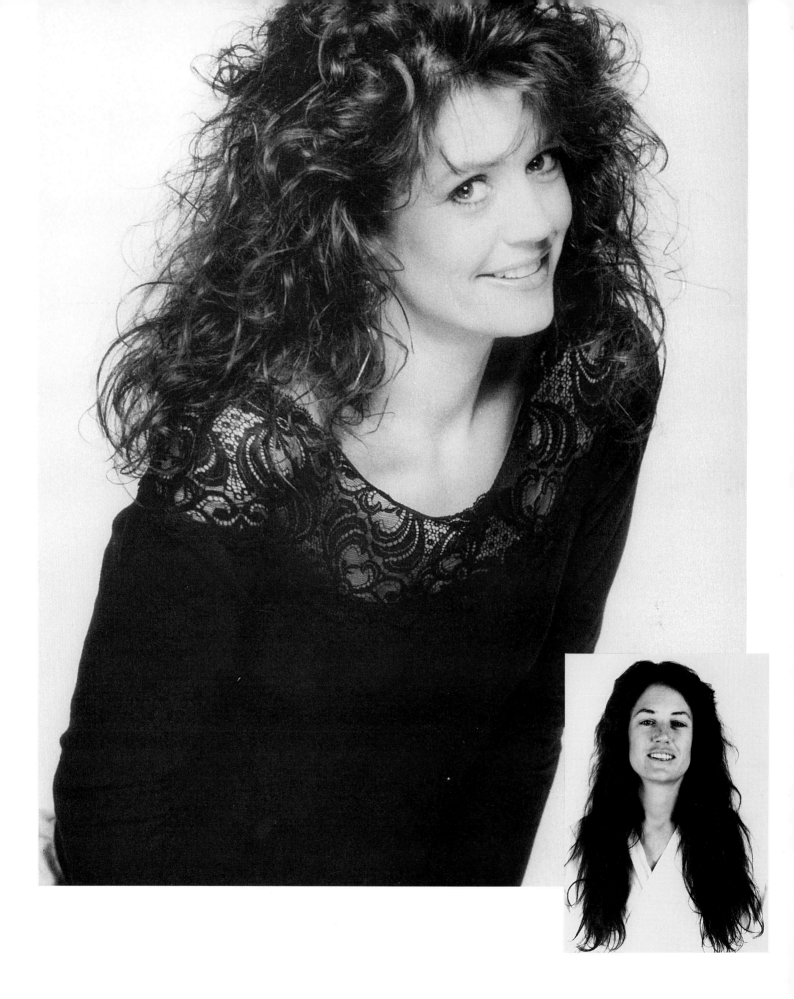

7

CREATING A DIVERSION

MOLLIE
RATTO

AGE: 31

OCCUPATION:
HOMEMAKER

PROBLEM:
WIDE JAW,
HIGH FOREHEAD

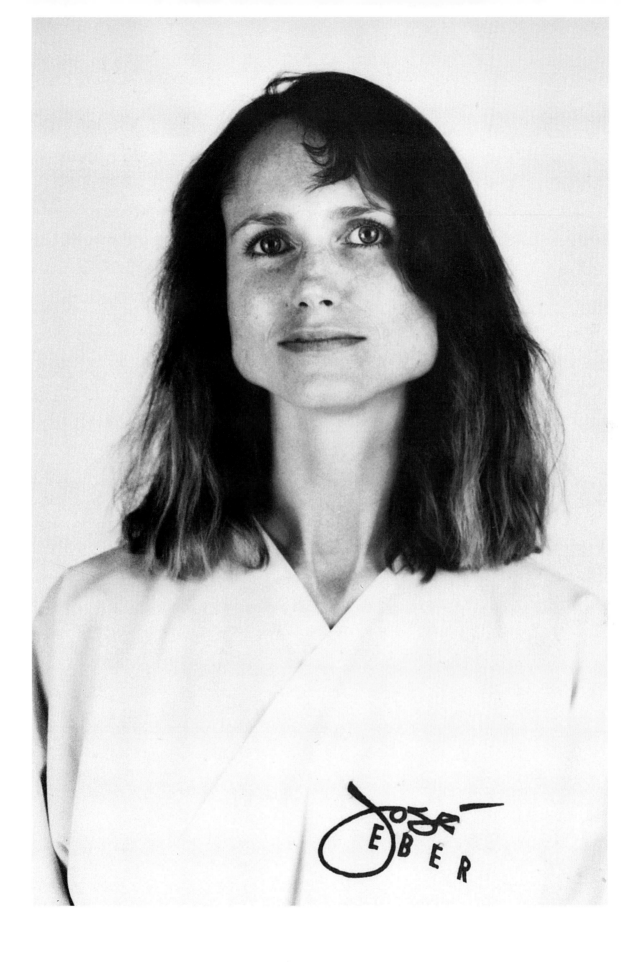

Mollie, a former ballerina, had just had her second child when she came to see me. All her attention had been focused on her children lately, and she felt she had let herself go a little. Personally I thought she looked fabulous, but if she didn't, I was certainly willing to help her improve the way she felt about herself.

With a new baby and a three-year-old in the house, Mollie needed above all else a style that would be easy to maintain. Yet I didn't want to sacrifice any of her femininity. Nor did I want to lose that sense of delicate strength that I saw at the heart of her attractiveness.

Mollie told me she was open to anything. She had no objection if I cut her hair short or changed its color. She just wanted to look alive again. What she didn't tell me was that, as she'd left her house that morning to come to the salon, her husband had made one request. "Please," he'd said to her, "whatever you do—don't let them dye your hair red."

Naturally, that was just the color we wound up selecting.

The most obvious thing about Mollie's face when I first met her was her pronounced jawline. It really detracted from her fabulous eyes. My goal was to create a style that would draw attention to those eyes. In order to do so, I cut her hair exactly to chin length and fringed it all around her face. Then I gave Mollie some light bangs, which de-emphasized her high forehead and highlighted her eyes. Sometimes, when you are trying to minimize certain parts of the face, it is better to create a diversion than to try to cover up what you might consider to be a flaw. In Mollie's case, I was able to hide her imperfections with a simple haircut.

Her hair color was somewhat uneven, dappled with leftover streaks from a previous coloring. Given Mollie's lightly freckled complexion and fair skin, I knew a rich, deep auburn would give her the lift she was after. I felt confident this was just the right shade to complete her new look. When I suggested it to Mollie she said fine, it sounded like fun to her.

When Mollie was finished, she really did look glamorous. I could tell she was happy because her whole face lit up—though when I suggested that she probably couldn't wait to get home and show her husband the new Mollie, she just looked at me kind of funny.

The key to making a style like Mollie's look good anytime is to have the right finger technique. All she has to do is get in there with her fingers and mess it up!

DOING IT YOURSELF

TOOLS NEEDED: Styling spritz, blow dryer, large round brush, curling iron (optional), hair spray.

You can re-create this look with practically no effort at all. After shampooing, squirt a little styling spritz onto your roots. Then tip your head upside down and blow your hair almost completely dry. After that, wrap the ends around a large round brush and continue with the blow dryer until all your hair has a soft, gentle bend to the ends. Then take your hands and mess up your hair, allowing it to fall back into place naturally, finishing it all with a bit of hair spray.

When you're not in a hurry, you can create a really special look by using a medium-size curling iron to give yourself lots of curls. But be warned, this is very time-consuming.

MOLLIE'S COMMENTS

The reaction from my family and friends has been totally positive—except, of course, that my husband is not big on red hair. Oh, well, you can't please everyone. He loves the cut, and I love both the cut and the color. And after all, it is *my* hair. Anyway, to tell you the truth, I think the color is growing on him.

As far as I'm concerned, there is far too much emphasis put on external appearances. Sure, it's fun to look your best. I think it's even good for you. But that's the thing—it's good for *you*. When I get my hair done or buy myself a new outfit, I do it for *me*.

Take my hair color. Of course, it's all been in good fun, but the fact remains that my husband doesn't particularly care for red hair. I, however, rather like the way it looks on me. So my hair is still red. The point is, the color of my hair shouldn't change the way my husband feels about me. And it doesn't.

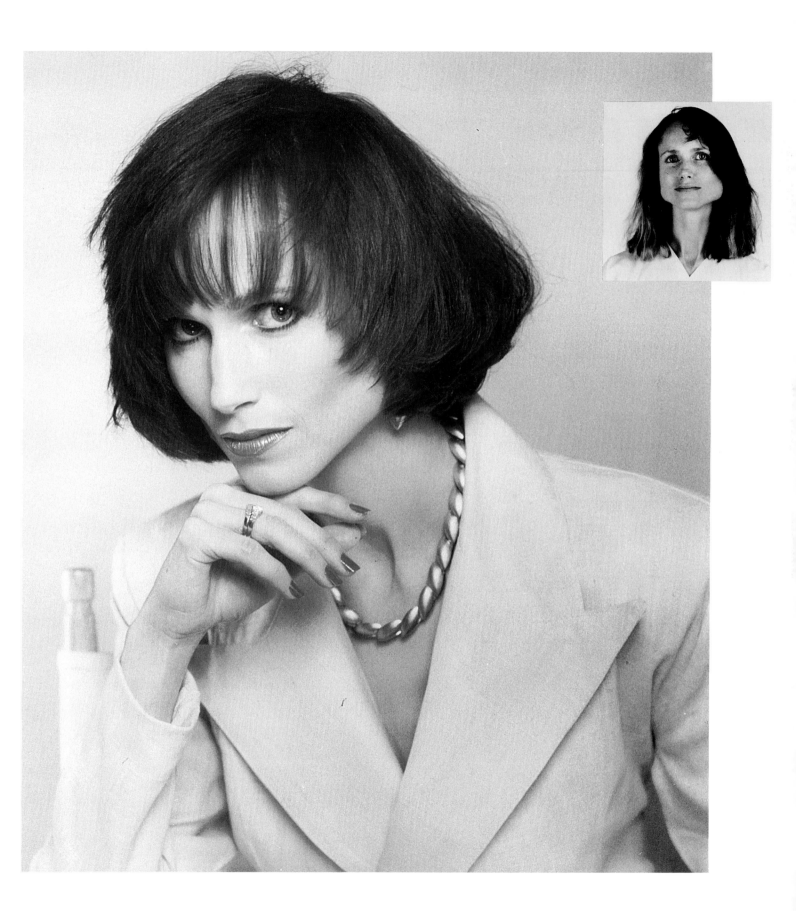

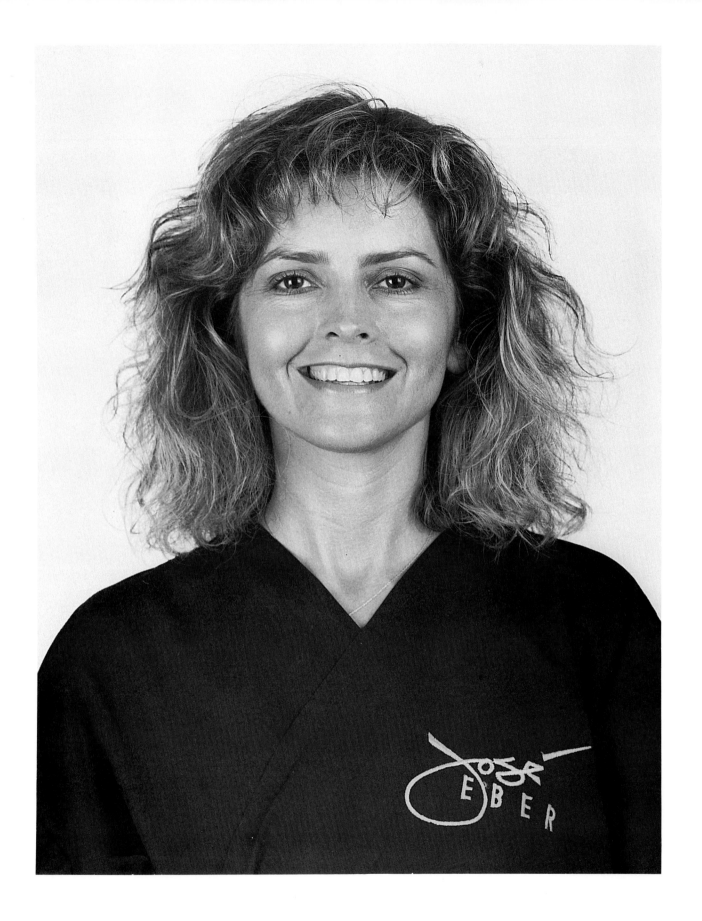

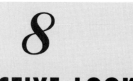

8

AN ACTIVE LOOK

DEBBIE
HENRY

AGE: 36

OCCUPATION:
EXERCISE
THERAPIST

PROBLEM:
OVERCOLORED,
DAMAGED HAIR

D E B B I E   H E N R Y

The first time I saw Debbie I thought she was very attractive. I know some of the other women who were in my salon at the time were wondering why she would want a makeover. I could feel it. So I asked her. "I want a new look," she replied. "I've tried everything to look different, and I always end up looking the same. I'm tired of it. I want a change."

To me, this proves a point I have always thought was true. It is very difficult to see ourselves as beautiful. A lot of women would like nothing better than to look like Debbie Henry. But she wants to look different. I'm not saying there is anything wrong with wanting to change the way you look, but I also wish we could be more self-accepting.

Debbie is very active. She and her husband, a top Los Angeles personal trainer, are committed to a healthy life-style. They teach individually during the day and then team up at night for even more exercise classes. I knew I had to find a look for Debbie that could keep up with her from dawn 'til way past dusk . . . .

o   o   o

The only problem I could see with Debbie was that her hair was damaged and the color was pretty dull and lifeless. It was sort of an interesting contrast. Here we had this fabulous-looking woman, the picture of health and vitality, with hair that could use a good workout. For years, she had been having it streaked with blond highlights. Although it had a good natural wave of its own, I discovered I was also seeing the remnants of an old perm.

When you meet Debbie she reminds you of a little ball of energy. I wanted her hair to reflect her effervescence. I didn't think her color was doing her justice, so after giving her hair a deep-conditioning treatment, I changed it to a lively shade of auburn. At once, she began to sparkle. The new color complemented her brown eyes and flattered her olive skin tone. Much the same as Oriental skin, olive skin has a tendency to appear a little yellow or greenish at times—especially when the skin is particularly pale or particularly tan. The problem can be corrected by using makeup foundation with a pink hue or a slightly rose-colored powder. But Debbie's daily workouts are not conducive to wearing cosmetics all the time. Besides, she looks terrific with auburn hair!

I didn't shorten her hair much at all. I just trimmed enough to remove the dead ends. Debbie had told me that, because of her athletic life-style, she wanted to leave her hair long enough to be able to pull it back away from her face.

Still, I knew that a style with a little more swing would give Debbie the younger, fresher look she was after. That's why I decided to blow her hair straight rather than allow it to dry with its natural wave. She loved it.

When your hair has body to it, as Debbie's does, sometimes it looks very chic to dry it straight as a stick. Although this doesn't work with stringy hair, look at the difference straight hair makes on Debbie. She finally looks like the young, vibrant woman she is *inside.*

This is another one of those fabulous cuts that requires almost no time to do at home. Debbie mastered it in minutes.

DOING IT YOURSELF

TOOLS NEEDED: Mousse, blow dryer, flat brush, large round brush, hair spray.

After shampooing, you apply a little mousse to your roots and tip your head upside down while blow-drying, using the flat brush in long even strokes. As your hair dries, the flat brush removes the curl. When your hair is completely dry, stand upright and bend the ends around your large round brush. This will give your hair just the slightest little curve. A bit of hair spray to keep your style in place and you're ready for the gym, the theater, or just a quiet evening at home.

DEBBIE'S COMMENTS

I had always wanted to be a Jose Eber makeover. I talked about it for years. I'd seen the miracles he'd performed on television and wondered what he could do for me. I was searching through the pages of every magazine trying to find a look that was right. Nothing seemed to work.

When I heard Jose was writing a book and looking for women to make over, I had to go down and see what it was all about. I told him of my frustrations, that I just felt I needed a change. He understood what I meant and said he could help.

I knew if anyone could give me a lift, it was Jose. And I was right. I don't think I would have ever thought of changing my color to auburn. It made me feel different. Believe it or not, it made me feel energized. That might sound like a silly thing to say about a hair color, but it's true. Blowing my hair straight gave me the polish and sophistication I had been lacking. A lot of people didn't recognize me at first, the change was so dramatic. But everyone loved it.

In order for other people to like you, *you* must like you. Sometimes we allow ourselves to get into ruts and become extremely bored. Boredom can disguise itself as self-hatred, making us think nothing is right in our lives. I know, it happened to me. The truth is I just needed a change. I had to step outside myself and look at myself objectively. I saw that my work had become routine. I had to do something to make it more interesting for me and those I work with. I also saw that I had been talking about making a change in my physical appearance for a long time without acting on it. If I wasn't boring people with the way I looked, I had to be boring people with the way I talked about it all the time. Or maybe I was just boring myself. Anyway, as a gift to me, I went to Jose for help. He gave me exactly what I needed—the knowledge that my life was pretty terrific all along.

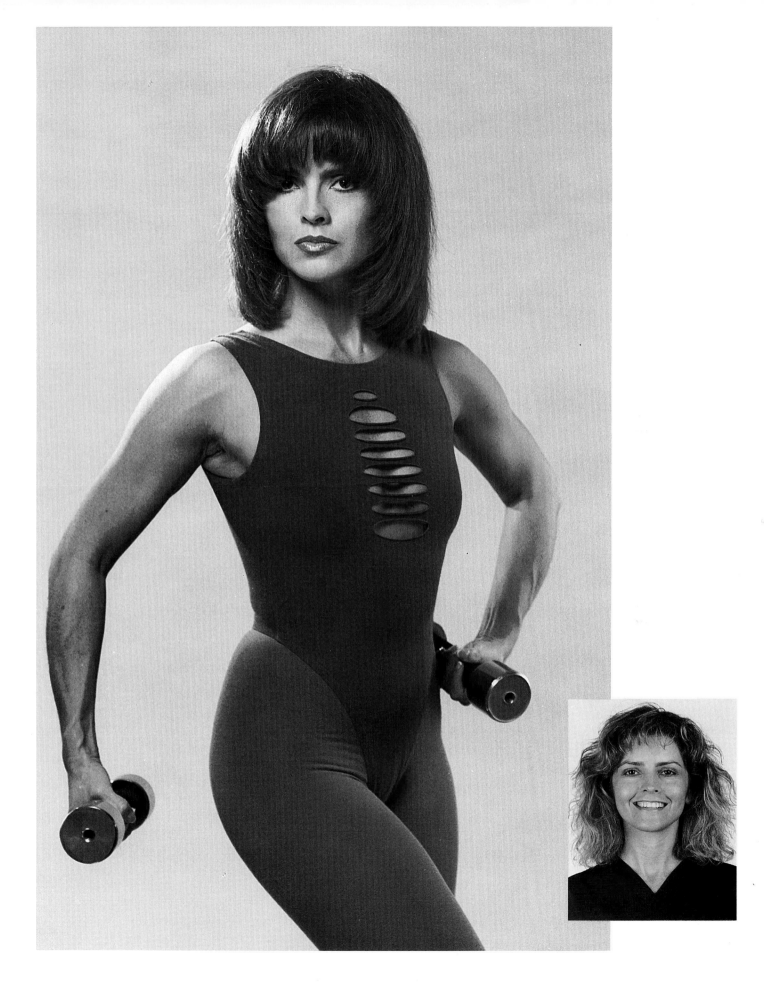

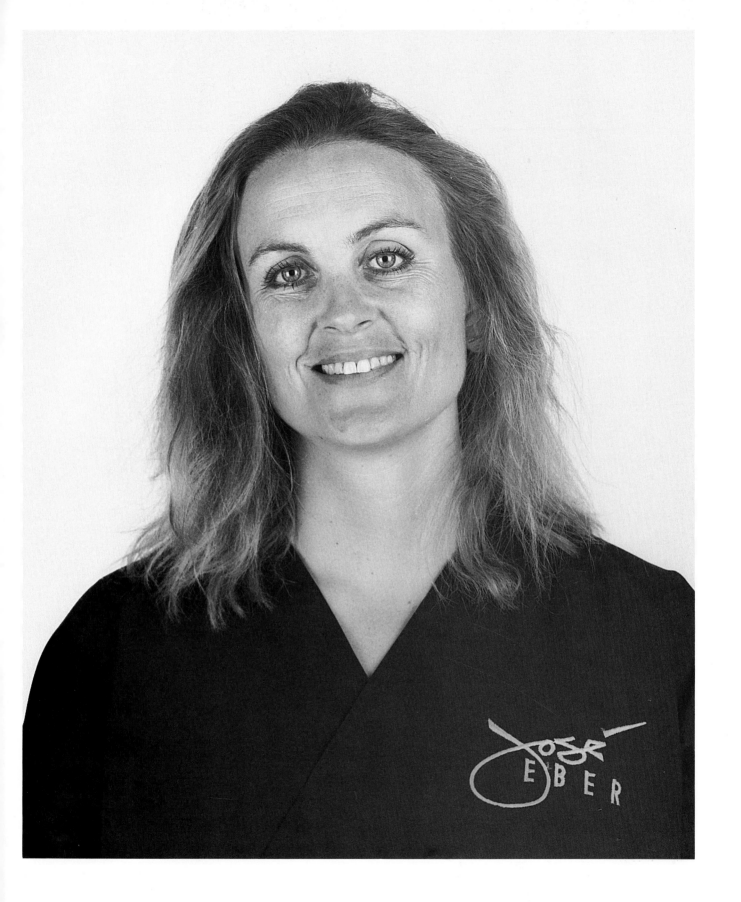

9

STYLING THE UNSTYLABLE

P A M   S H A W

AGE: 36

OCCUPATION:
COSTUME DESIGNER

PROBLEM:
THIN, FINE HAIR;
HEAD NOT IN
PROPORTION TO BODY

P A M   S H A W

The first time I saw Pam I thought she was striking. Standing six feet tall, she commands attention right away. Yet she is still decidedly feminine. When I asked Pam what she wanted to change about the way she looked, she said her hair was unstylable. She had had no luck with cuts, no luck with color, no luck with perms. Her hair simply would not hold a style. Usually, the only way to make it look decent was to pull it back in a knot or chignon. Though she was dying for a look that was different, she had just about given up trying.

I felt challenged by Pam's dilemma. I saw no reason why this already pretty woman couldn't look and feel the way she wanted to. It is horribly frustrating when you can picture yourself looking a certain way but not know how to achieve it. I think it is especially so when you are a very creative person like Pam, who makes her living designing costumes for film, theater, and television. In a sense, Pam does for the body what I do for the head. She could give everyone the look they wanted—except herself.

What I first noticed about Pam was that her head was out of proportion with the rest of her body. Pam is tall and has a fairly large bone structure. In comparison, her head is very small. Her thin, flat hair made it look even smaller. I knew that if I could give her hair more volume, more excitement on top, her head would seem larger.

To add volume, I layered her hair, making sure to keep the layers long. Pam enjoys being able to wear her hair completely off her face, and I didn't want to take that pleasure away from her. Still, I felt that should be an option, rather than the only thing she could do with her hair. That meant leaving her hair long enough to give Pam the flexibility to be able to change her style when and if she desired.

Given how fine her hair is, the only way to provide Pam with the kind of body and volume she needs to maintain a style is with a permanent wave. We gave her a very unconstructed spiral perm that instantly made her hair look fuller, longer, and healthier. The beauty of the perm is that Pam can have this fullness and body from the moment she wakes up until she goes to sleep—without ever having to work at it.

For the finishing touch, I decided to warm Pam up with a little bit of nonperoxide color. I wasn't looking for drama, but rather a blending of all her previous coloring attempts as well as the natural bleaching of the sun. I used a very light mahogany shade that brought out the gold in Pam's complexion.

The truth is, we did a lot to Pam's hair—we cut it, we permed it, and we colored it. But the results were certainly worth the effort. Her hair has more style and energy than ever before. And Pam looks fabulous!

DOING IT YOURSELF

TOOLS NEEDED: Mousse, gel, comb or pick, blow dryer, diffuser, curling iron (optional), hair spray.

This look takes a little more time than some of the others to achieve at home. After shampooing, you add mousse to your roots. Then comb out the tangles with a pick or comb. Next, apply a small amount of gel to the rest of your hair in order to add weight and prevent frizzing. To prevent your hair from losing its wave and becoming frizzy, you must use a diffuser in conjunction with the blow dryer. After your hair is completely dry, use a curling iron on the top and around the face for even more lift and body. For every day, you may want to skip the curling iron and wear a softer wave. Using your fingers, pull your hair up at the roots for height and push the hair into place with your hands before finishing with a little hair spray.

Notice the proportion of Pam's head to her body in her "after" photos compared with the "before" photos. She appears much more balanced and even as a result of the added volume and fullness on top. Pam was pretty to begin with, but now she looks glamorous and together and sexy. And Pam thought it couldn't be done.

PAM'S COMMENTS

I had tried everything to make my hair look better, and nothing seemed to help. Although I had seen Jose work wonders on television, I just didn't think he could do it for me. Not because he wasn't terrific, but because my hair wasn't. I'm glad I decided to give it one more try.

I get very angry when I see how much emphasis is placed on the way people look rather than the way people are. It is especially difficult for women. Magazines and television always seem to show women as gorgeous, scantily clad sexpots—whether they're in the bedroom, the kitchen, the nursery, or the boardroom. That just isn't reality. When men see this and then look at their wives or girlfriends, they become disappointed. When women see this and then look in the mirror, *they* become disappointed. I don't understand why the media can't show women the way they really are. Sometimes we look good, and sometimes we don't. Sure, we'd all like to look our best all the time, but most women simply can't.

Jose is helping to change that. He neither expects physical perfection nor strives for it. He just wants his clients to feel good about the way they present themselves. I respect that. There is something very enjoyable about feeling your best and looking your best. By the same token, there is something very pathetic about desperately trying to look perfect all the time.

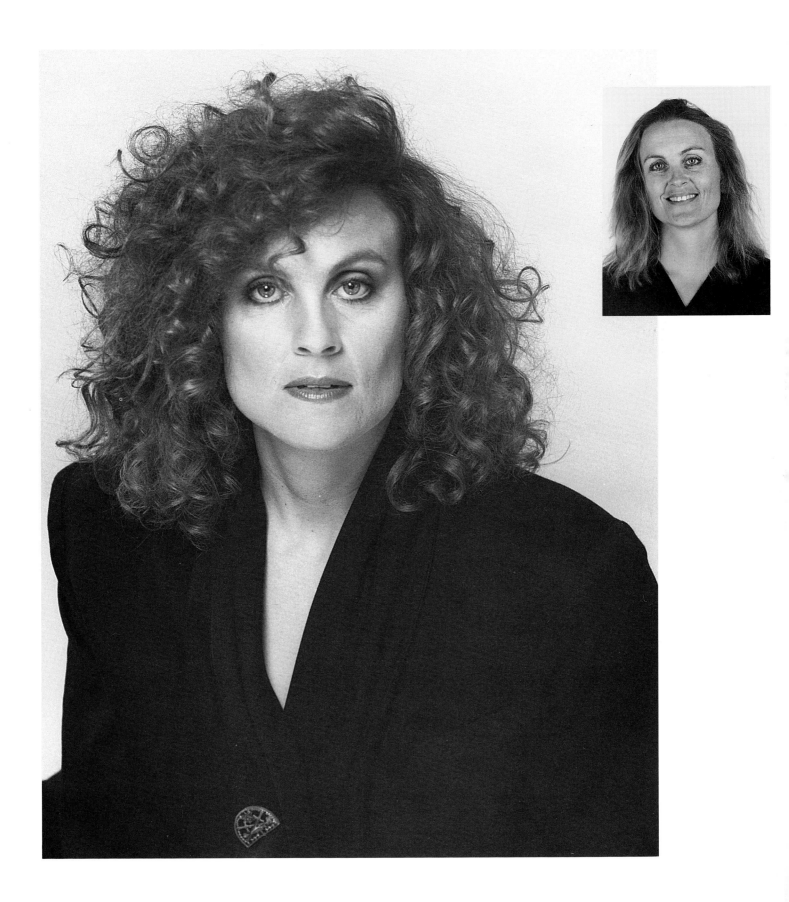

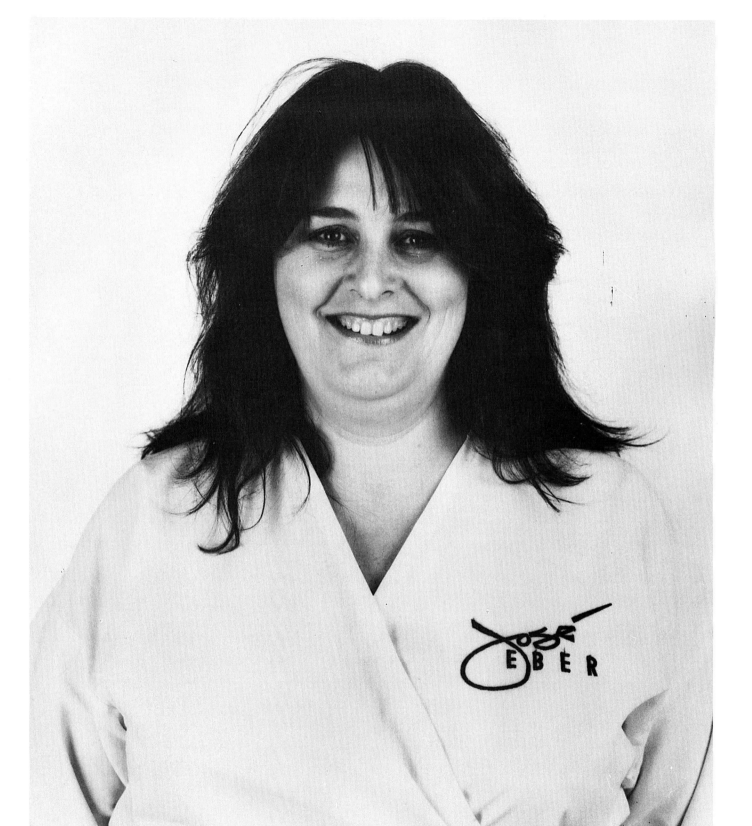

10

BIG CAN BE BEAUTIFUL

CATHERINE

KENNEDY

AGE: 37

CAREER:

EXECUTIVE

ASSISTANT

PROBLEM:

FULL FACE,

DOUBLE CHIN

C A T H E R I N E   K E N N E D Y

I have never read any law that says a woman has to be a size four to be beautiful. When I go to the museum and look at the paintings of the women men dreamed of, I don't see any skinny figures. All the women portrayed in those pictures had full, round figures. And they were adored.

Still, we're not living in Rubens's day. These are the 1990s, and the reality is that it's *unhealthy* to be overweight. *That's* the reason to keep your weight in line. It shouldn't be because you're obsessed with looking like the models in your favorite magazines or that you live in fear of being publicly humiliated by insensitive strangers.

When I met Catherine, she had come to a major turning point in her life. After years of pain and torment, she had decided, once and for all, to take off her extra weight. When I asked her why she was going on a diet and why she thought this one would work, she told me that this time she was doing it for herself. Not to please her husband, a boyfriend, or a family member. Well, maybe one family member. Catherine is the mother of an eight-year-old boy, Carroll. Though Carroll loves her just the way she is, Catherine realized that in order to get the most out of their relationship, she had to be in good health. A divorcée, she raises her son alone. "I've got to be healthy," she explained. "Carroll needs me."

Going on a diet wasn't the only thing happening in Catherine's life when we met. She was also in the process of making a career change. I loved the fact that she was taking action in order to improve the quality of her life. I really wanted to help. . . .

o o o

There is a quality about Catherine that I truly admire. Many women say, "I'll get a makeover after I lose the weight," or, "I'll change jobs as soon as I get thin. Then my life will be happy." Catherine didn't say that at all. What she said to herself was, "I'm going to start improving the quality of my life today." Her determined spirit reminded me of Oprah Winfrey. Oprah didn't wait until she got thin to become successful. She got thin in order to get more pleasure from her success. Oprah insisted that people accept her the way she was. And you know what? They did. The same thing is going to happen for Catherine. I can feel it.

Looking at her, I could see Catherine looked a bit lopsided. Her body was large, but her hair was thin and flat. In order to give her some balance and to draw attention to her face, I cut her hair in a lot more layers. Of course, layering will only make hair look fuller when it has a lot of body, when there is a wave or curls that can frame the face. Unfortunately, Catherine's hair lacked body and volume. To compensate, I gave her a body wave for fullness.

As I mentioned earlier, a body wave is a perm that is wound on very large rods and timed so that the result is wavy, not curly. It can be a godsend to people with straight, fine locks, making their hair instantly appear thicker, coarser, and healthier. In short, it creates the illusion of "bigger" hair.

That's certainly what it did for Catherine. Right away, her silhouette became more even.

Was it our imagination, or did Catherine look thinner? What happened was that she *felt* pretty. As a result, she stood taller, held her chin up, and looked at herself with kindlier eyes.

To re-create this style at home, Catherine will need a few extra minutes in the morning. Since she enjoys fooling around with her hair, the additional time is no problem.

DOING IT YOURSELF

TOOLS NEEDED: Mousse, blow dryer, diffuser, hot rollers, hair spray.

Once again, for a little extra body with this style, add mousse to your roots after shampooing. Because of the body wave, it is important that you use a diffuser on your blow dryer to avoid frizziness. When your hair is completely dry, curl it away from your face using large-size hot rollers. This will give you a gentle curl rather than the wave of a perm. After removing the rollers, flip on your blow dryer again (this time without the diffuser since your hair is already dry) and stretch out those curls with your fingers. Then add a bit of hair spray to keep the style in place, and you are ready to go.

CATHERINE'S COMMENTS

I grew up in Virginia and watched Jose religiously on television. I guess you could say I worshiped him from afar. I can't remember how many times I fantasized about him coming into my life and making me beautiful. In my dreams, Jose would not only make my hair look fabulous, but he would make me thin, too. Once I came to visit my sister in Los Angeles, and while I was visiting I called Jose's Beverly Hills salon and tried to make an appointment. I was heartbroken when they said he was all booked up and couldn't see me. I went home again and continued dreaming.

When I moved here with my little boy eight years later, I was determined to turn fantasy into reality. Imagine my delight when I heard that Jose was looking for all kinds of women to put in his new book. I thought I'd die if I wasn't chosen. Fortunately, my life was spared.

Jose was exactly how I thought he would be—warm, funny, sensitive, and caring. Let's face it. Walking into Jose Eber's beauty salon could have been a disaster for a woman as overweight as me. But something inside told me not to worry, it would be okay. It was. I told him about my diet and my reasons for sticking to it. I also told him about my new job and the plans I had for the future. It honestly mattered to him, and I was thrilled.

When you are dramatically overweight, life can be hell. You try not to look at yourself, if possible, and are always disappointed when it can't be avoided. You pray every day that you can get through a crowd without being laughed at, and God forbid you make a mistake in the car. Apparently, fat drivers are much worse than thin drivers. No other humiliation compares with going clothes shopping—unless, that is, the unthinkable happens and some horrible human being suggests going to the beach. Life as a fat person can be pretty awful. People understand drug addicts, they even understand alcoholics, but they don't understand food addicts. Every

Monday morning I would put myself on a diet, but I never made it past lunch on Tuesday. I needed help.

Today, I'm much more settled. I discovered the *reason* I was overeating and tackled that problem first. If you are a drug addict, you can get off drugs and never touch them again. When you quit drinking alcohol, you can live the rest of your life without it. But when your addiction is food, you simply have to learn to control it. After all, you can't live without food.

Starting this diet has given me a new lease on life. Every single day I know I'm on the road to better health. Instead of waiting until I'm thin to enjoy my life, I am determined to enjoy the process.

Jose was the first person I spoke to about all of these new thoughts. He told me I had inner beauty. It was a powerful blending of emotions when my fantasy met reality. Yes, Jose made me feel beautiful, but no, he didn't make me thin. He did, however, applaud my effort to do it myself, and *that* meant even more.

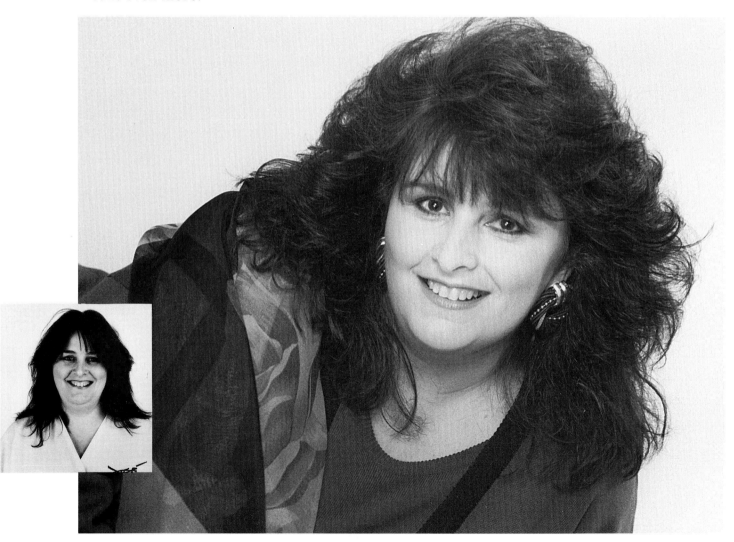

11

SOFTENING STRONG FEATURES

SANDRA MILLER

AGE: 37

**OCCUPATION:
WRITER**

**PROBLEM:
WIDE NOSE,
WIDE JAW,
STRONG FEATURES**

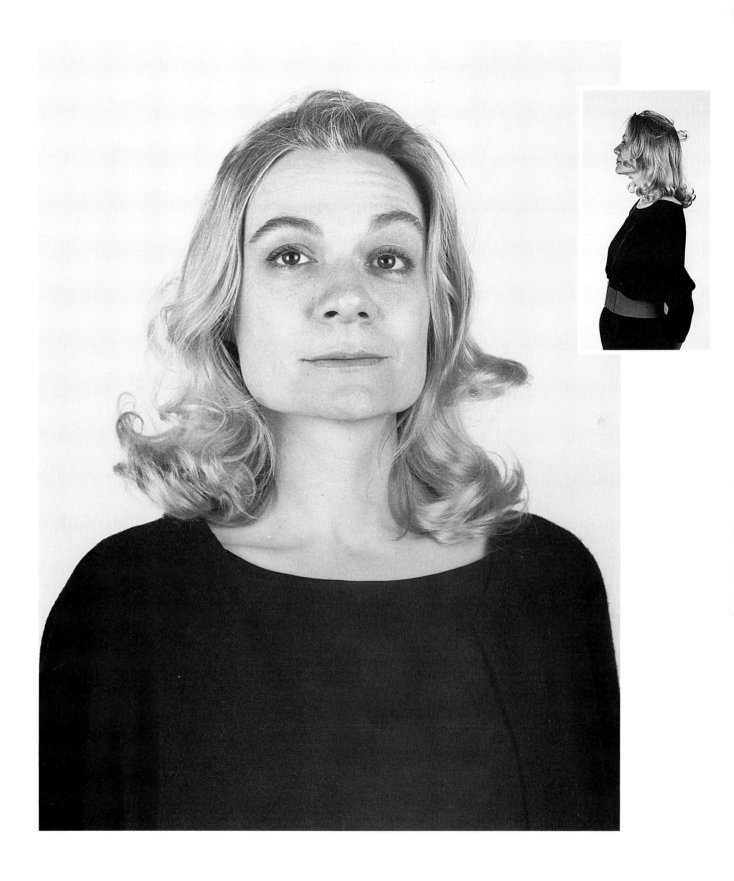

S A N D R A   M I L L E R

Sandra Miller is not the sort of woman who should walk into a room and go unnoticed. She is nearly six feet tall, very statuesque, and sort of glides by you with an air of mystery. Yet the night I met her, she seemed not to want to be noticed at all. It made me wonder why she had come to my salon. When I asked her, Sandra told me she was tired of the same old look she had had for years. She wanted to look different but didn't know where to begin. Maybe shorten her hair, but not too short. Maybe a color change, but not too dark. She wanted to wear makeup, but not too much.

I knew she didn't feel as though she looked her best, and that made me sad. I felt that with a few changes she could look fabulous. The minute I saw Sandra I had some ideas I thought would help. But before I could act on those ideas, I had to take a few minutes to talk to her about her life-style. I had to know what kind of time constraints she had in her day and how much she enjoyed fiddling with her hair and face.

I discovered that Sandra is a writer who does a lot of her work at home, so she has more time to devote to herself than someone who is on the go a lot. I also discovered that she used to be an actress and acting coach. No wonder she wasn't satisfied—Sandra needed a little drama in her appearance!

The first thing that jumped out at me about Sandra's face was her pronounced jaw and strong nose. That was because all the activity in her hair was happening around her chin, which drew my attention directly to her jaw. To make matters worse, her hair color was the same tone as her skin—there was no contrast at all. This made Sandra look washed-out and ashen. I knew that if I provided some contrast by darkening her hair color, it would brighten up her face immediately. Indeed, the first thing everyone noticed when we changed her hair from blond to toast was the amazing hazel of Sandra's eyes. It was funny because no one commented on her beautiful eyes until after the color change.

The haircut made a huge difference. I got rid of a lot of length on the sides but kept it longer on the neck. Adding lots of layers gave Sandra a more feminine feeling, which really helped soften her strong features. What's more, giving her height on top diverted attention from her jaw to her eyes. We also suggested that she wear large earrings in order to bring the focus to the sides of her face rather than the middle.

It was hard to believe that the Sandra Miller who walked into my salon was the same Sandra Miller who walked out of my salon. On the day of the photo session it was just like watching a *Vogue* model in action. Everyone was talking about how great she looked and the dramatic change that had taken place. Sandra seemed more surprised than anyone. Frankly, it didn't surprise me a bit. I knew she had it in her all the time.

This is a style that takes a bit of practice to get the hang of at first. But the end result is worth the effort.

DOING IT YOURSELF

TOOLS NEEDED: Mousse, styling spritz, blow dryer, vent brush, large curling iron or large hot rollers, hair spray.

After shampooing, you apply both mousse and styling spritz to your roots. If you have a lot of natural wave to your hair, you will only need one or the other. Then bend over and, vent brush in hand, blow-dry your hair until it is completely dry. After that, use a large curling iron and roll your hair, one small section at a time, away from your face. When all your hair is rolled, pull your bangs forward and stretch the curl with your fingers. A small amount of teasing on the top followed by a bit of hair spray, and this style is completed!

Some women find it easier to work with hot rollers than a curling iron. This style works equally well with either. If you decide to use hot rollers, be sure to use the largest size.

SANDRA'S COMMENTS

When I first walked into the Jose Eber salon and saw all those women waiting for Jose to look them over, I almost turned and walked out. But I decided, What the heck. I've driven all the way over, I might as well hear what the man has to say. I was surprised when he didn't say anything at first. He wanted to listen to what *I* thought about what I needed. For some reason I just assumed an expert like Jose would take charge and tell me what I should have done. Instead, he wanted us to decide together.

When I walked into Jose's salon I felt like I had the weight of the world on my shoulders. When I walked out I felt fun and carefree and giddy.

It is difficult to tell if a person is beautiful these days. It seems like everyone is wearing the same uniform. No one wants to be different. Is the need to be accepted so great that we are willing to freely give up our individuality for it? To me, that's too high a price to pay. And what about those of us doing the accepting? Are we so insecure that we must ostracize a person just because she looks different? What ever happened to all the great eccentrics, those who are brave enough to set the trends rather than follow them?

In order to have inner beauty a person must have enough self-love and self-interest to enjoy her own company when no one else is around. Yet she must also be genuinely concerned about people other than herself. It is a rare combination I have had the pleasure of seeing only a few times.

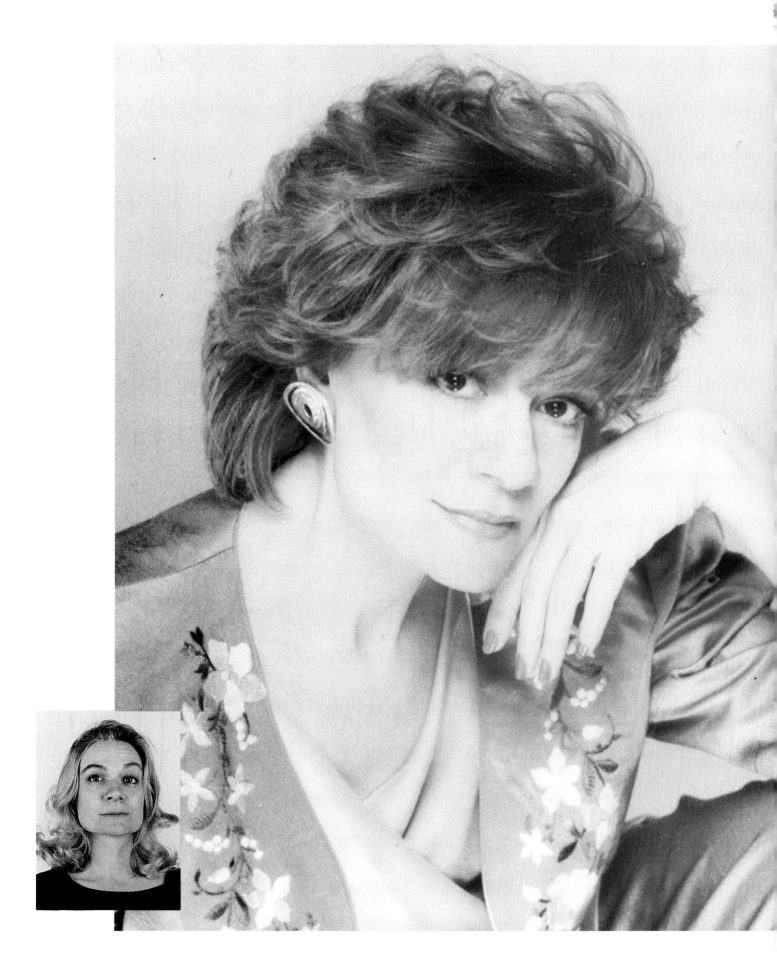

12

A BEANPOLE BLOSSOMS

FAYE BELAND

AGE: 38

OCCUPATION:

INTERNATIONAL FILM DISTRIBUTOR

PROBLEM:

VERY THIN FACE, LOW FOREHEAD

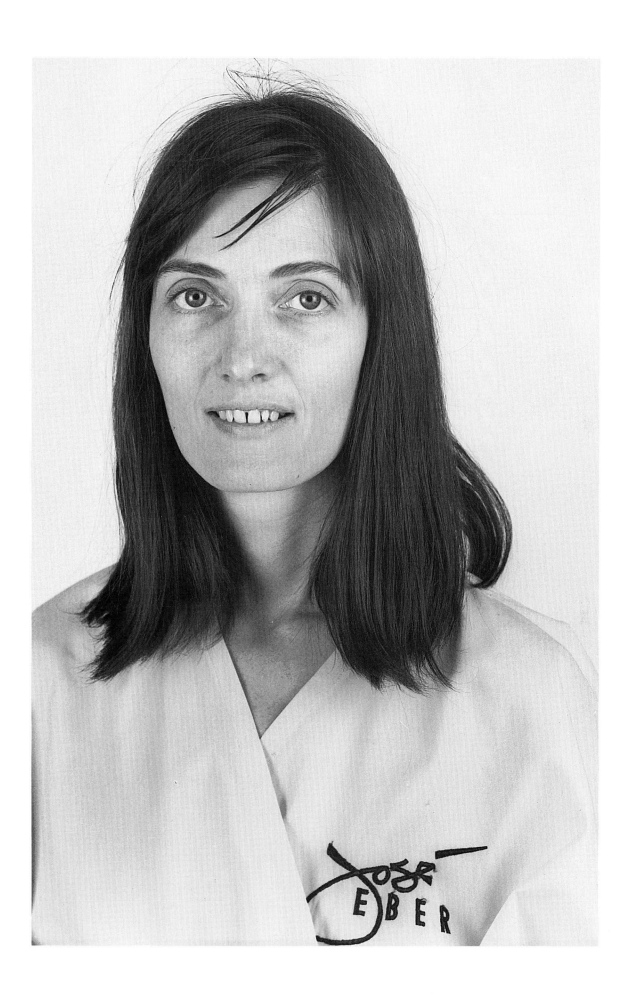

FAYE BELAND

The first time I met Faye, she reminded me of Greta Garbo. Of course, I don't think anyone else saw the potential, least of all Faye herself. She stood there in my salon, looking shy and rather uncomfortable. I walked up and asked her what she felt her problems were, what she would like to change about the way she looked. "Well," she said, "I need something. My hair is so straight and dull. Actually, I would love a whole new image." There was something in Faye's eyes that told me, yes, she was ready for a change. Not just in the way she looked, but in the way she felt about herself. I could sense that she had been through some pain and was ready to let it go and move ahead with her life. I wanted to help.

In talking with Faye, I discovered that she was a single, working mother who lived with her four-year-old daughter. Although this told me that she had a limited amount of free time, I could also see that Faye had a very feminine way about her, that she enjoyed being a lady and wouldn't mind fussing over herself a little bit. As an international film distributor, Faye found herself traveling to Europe and other parts of the world quite often. That meant she had to have a look that was totally chic. At the same time, however, I knew she wouldn't want to carry around a lot of supplies and appliances in her suitcase.

The first thing people used to notice when they looked at Faye was that she was tall and skinny. Even though most women say they would kill for a body like hers, for Faye her thinness was a problem. Wearing her hair long and stick straight the way she did only accentuated that "beanpole" look. Her hair looked just like her body.

By Faye's own admission, the color of her hair was dull and lifeless. I can't tell you how many women have described their hair to me like that over the years. What was wrong with Faye's hair was that it was ordinary. It had no shine, no luster, nothing that made you want to touch it or feel it. I wanted to give her hair some sparkle and pizzazz! Given her fair skin, I decided on a light shade of auburn. When a woman has a white, porcelain-doll complexion, shades of auburn and copper are almost always appropriate because they look authentic. It is an especially believable choice if the woman is as freckled as Faye.

I cut Faye's hair in a chin-length bob to break the vertical look she had before. I let her keep her bangs, but I started them from much farther back, almost all the way back to the crown of her head, to give her the illusion of a higher forehead. I'm not saying that everyone must have a high forehead. Sometimes a high forehead is the problem. The point is, your forehead should be in proper proportion to the rest of your face. Faye's low forehead was not in proportion because the rest of her face was so long. By cutting her bangs the way I did, her face appeared much more even and centered.

There is nothing complicated or difficult about this style. It was easy for Faye to re-create, and it will be easy for you, too, if this is the style you and your hairdresser decide is right for you.

DOING IT YOURSELF

TOOLS NEEDED: Styling spritz, blow dryer, large round brush, hair spray.

To maintain this look at home, all you need are a few minutes in the morning. After shampooing, you towel-dry your hair, then spray the styling spritz near the roots for extra body. Then bend over and with your hair hanging down, begin to blow-dry it. Drying your hair upside down leaves it seeming thicker and fuller. After a few minutes, straighten up and wrap the ends of your hair around a large, round brush and finish blow-drying. Rather than a real curly look, this gives the hair a softer, gentler curve. Use the same technique on your bangs. You finish with a couple of squirts of hair spray and—voilà!

FAYE'S COMMENTS

Beauty is a state of mind. I never knew how true a statement that was until now. The week before I met Jose, my ex-husband got remarried. I was feeling so low and unattractive. I was sure that no one would ever look at me again. Why his getting married made me ugly, I don't know. But that's how I felt. I knew I had to do something. I started to focus on the good things in my life—my daughter, my job, my friends and family. I realized I was better off than a lot of other people. It dawned on me that his getting married was simply an end to a chapter. And when one chapter ends, another one begins. I needed to get ready for the new chapter.

I know that even at my best I don't fit into the conventional standard of beauty. I'm different. Jose helped me to realize that doesn't mean I'm not beautiful. He made me believe that looking different wasn't bad. I have never felt as secure and comfortable with myself as I do today. Jose didn't make me beautiful, he showed me that I already was.

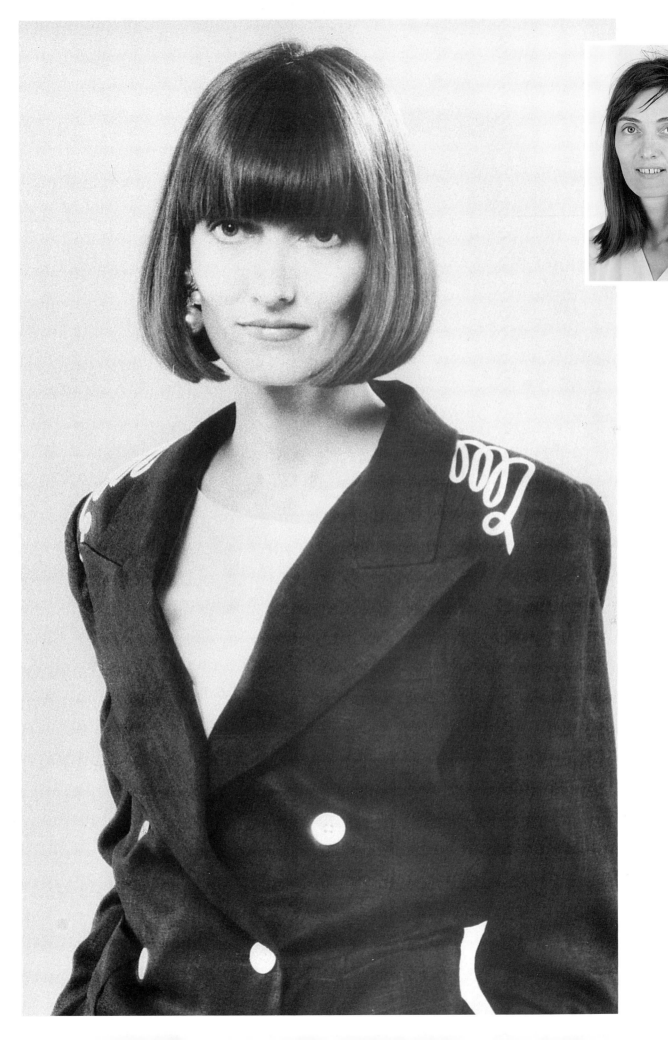

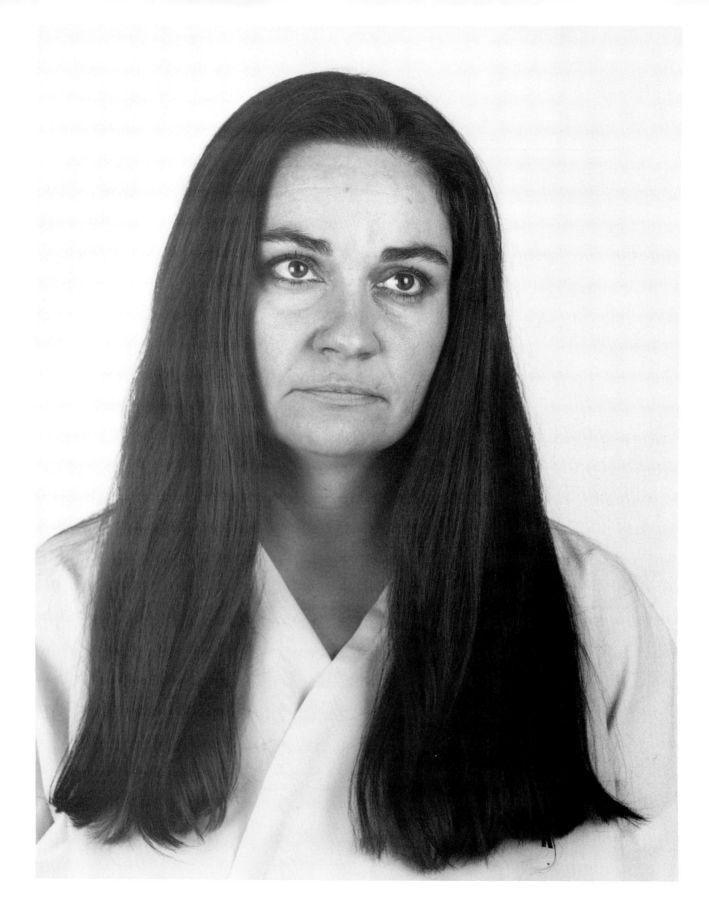

13

LEAVING THE SIXTIES BEHIND

KAREN GARGEL

AGE: 38

OCCUPATION:

KINDERGARTEN

TEACHER

PROBLEM:

FULL, SAD FACE;

NO STYLE TO

HAIR

K A R E N   G A R G E L

When Karen first walked into my salon, I was struck by how sad she
looked. I thought she was unhappy about something and went over to ask
her what was wrong. As it turned out, Karen was fine. She wasn't sad
about anything at all. As a matter of fact, she seemed pretty content and
cheerful. Karen said she had come in because she hadn't changed her
appearance in years and thought it was time to do something about it. She
wore her hair long, straight, and parted down the middle, a holdover from
the sixties. Karen admitted that's exactly how long she'd had the same
style. I agreed it was time for a change.

In talking with Karen, I got the impression that she was a fairly conservative woman who would feel most comfortable with a traditional look.
Still, I knew we could update her appearance and make her feel younger
and more in style. I also knew that spending all day with a roomful of
children was enough to drain anyone's energy, so whatever we did to
Karen's hair had to be easy for her to maintain at home. I saw something
in her eyes that told me she is a gentle, kind-hearted woman. I wanted that
to reflect in her whole face. . . .

Karen has beautiful hair. She was born with it. It's thick, healthy, and
shiny. Obviously she has taken very good care of it over the years. Unfortunately, in trying to avoid damaging her hair, Karen resisted making any
changes at all. As a result, she looked older than she needed to look.

There used to be a sort of unwritten law that women over thirty should
not wear their hair long. I think that's ridiculous. But no matter how old
she is, a woman with long hair must keep it in an up-to-date style. If she

doesn't, it's as if she's wearing a sign around her neck that says, "I'm as old as my hairstyle." The fact is, wearing a sixties-style hairdo doesn't make you look as young as you were in the sixties.

So the first thing I did to Karen's hair was cut it a bit shorter, bringing it up to her shoulders. That automatically eliminated the weight that made her face look droopy and sad. The next thing I did was to add a few layers around the sides and on top to give her a more feminine feeling. That made her face brighten up instantly. Almost all the activity in her hair now fell right around her dimples—dimples that I'll bet no one noticed before.

Coloring was simple. Though Karen's hair had a lot of gray in it, there wasn't enough for a great salt-and-pepper look. So we simply took it all out. We left her color the same rich mixture of cocoa shades that it had been to begin with—only now it's minus all the gray.

These small changes turned the sad-faced Karen Gargel who walked into my salon into a younger, fresher, vibrant-looking woman. And to maintain this new look, Karen will have to spend only a few minutes of her valuable time.

DOING IT YOURSELF

TOOLS NEEDED: Mousse, blow dryer, vent brush, hot rollers, hair spray.

You start by applying a little mousse to your roots after shampooing. Then tip your head upside down and blow-dry your hair completely. Next you curl your hair with large-size hot rollers, letting it all sit for a few minutes while you apply your makeup. After removing the hot rollers, turn your head upside down again and brush out some of the curl, leaving your hair full of body. If you like, you can tease your hair a little at the roots for extra lift. I'm not talking about the kind of teasing we practiced in the sixties, but a softer, more isolated form of teasing that really helps hard-to-hold areas. I teased Karen's hair, and it didn't look unnatural at all. With a few squirts of hair spray, Karen's style will last all day long and into the night. She can go from the kindergarten classroom to a teacher's meeting to a dinner date without ever worrying about her hair. And knowing she looks terrific!

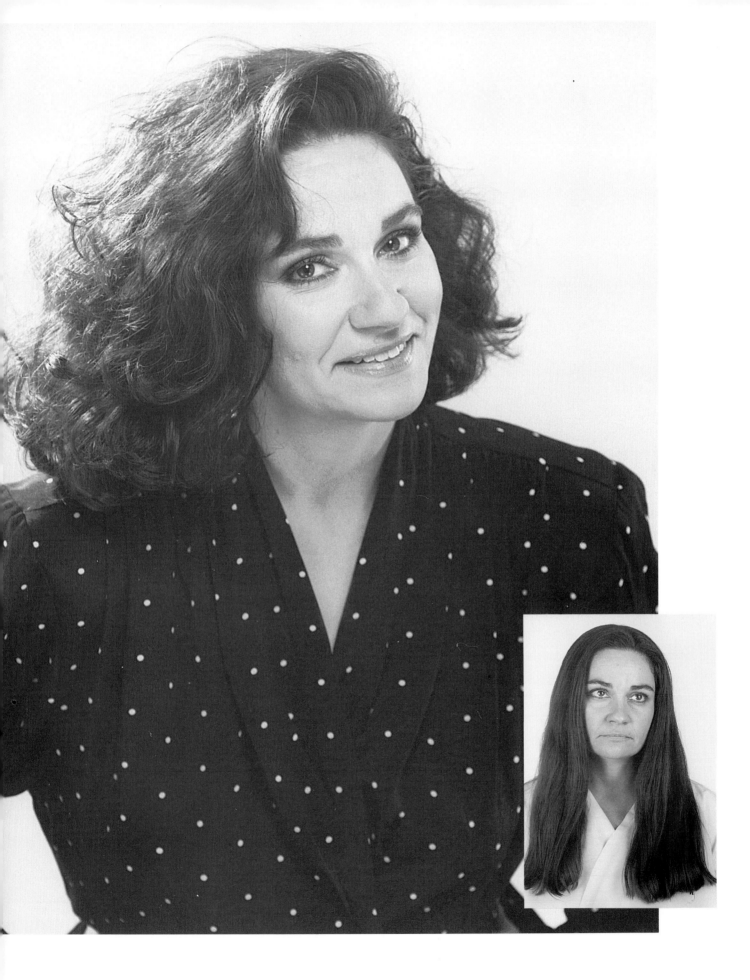

KAREN'S COMMENTS

I had thought about having Jose do my hair for a long time. I even went so far as to call the television station one day where he was doing a live appearance, after seeing the miracles he performed on a couple of women. But I got nervous and hung up.

Being made over was a little scary. After all, I hadn't done *anything* to my hair in years. The positive changes were infectious, though, and with every passing minute I felt better about myself.

People have said I look younger, that I seem energized, that I've lost weight, and that I've had a change in attitude. Well, I have! I feel great.

It's a wonderful feeling to know you look your best. Whether your best is beautiful or not is strictly in the eye of the beholder. Beauty is such an ethereal concept, who's to say if someone is beautiful? All we can go by is our own opinions. Maybe blind people know better than anyone. It seems to me that if we are going to judge beauty, we should do it without ever looking at a person's face or body.

To me, inner beauty comes from the confidence you get from being loved and knowing you've been the kind of person who deserves love. Raising children in a loving family is the best way to nurture inner beauty at a young age.

I wish I could make the children I see every day understand that *looking at a person with outer beauty is pleasurable, but looking at a person with inner beauty is joyous.* Unfortunately, that is something they'll have to learn all by themselves.

14

REJUVENATING EXHAUSTED HAIR

JOHNETTA BUSH

AGE: 40

OCCUPATION:
ADMINISTRATIVE
ASSISTANT/
SINGER

PROBLEM:
OVERRELAXED
HAIR,
VERY ROUND FACE

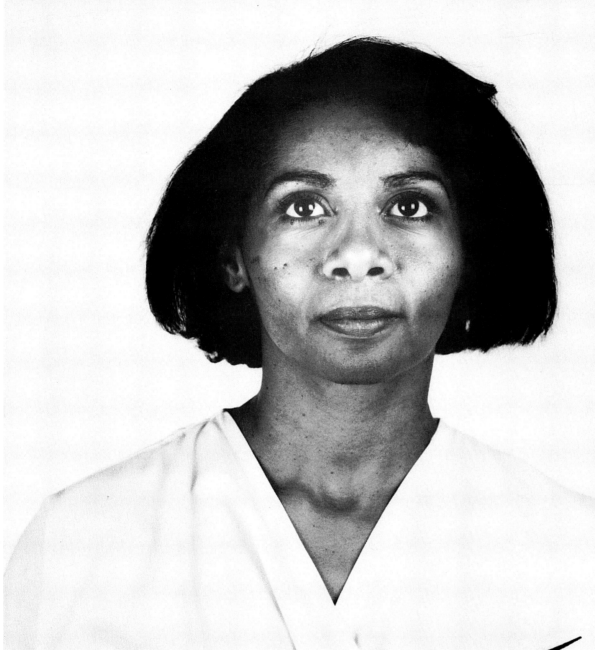

JOHNETTA BUSH

When I looked at Johnetta the first time, I knew that I could make her look gorgeous. She had incredible facial features and the potential for real beauty. When I told this to her, she looked at me as if to say, "Prove it!" She said she had tried everything to make her hair look decent and nothing worked. I told her that was just the problem. She had done too much of everything. Johnetta's hair was overprocessed, overrelaxed, overworked. Her hair was exhausted, and it showed. As a matter of fact, it gave her whole appearance a sort of tired, lifeless feeling.

Still, there was a certain twinkle in Johnetta's eye that told me this woman had a lot of life in her. After a little chat, I learned that although Johnetta was working as an administrative assistant for a commercial loan company, her real aspiration was to become a professional singer. She needed the look of a confident, secure entertainer. Because Johnetta sings a lot of gospel, pop, and jazz music, I knew the rock star image wouldn't do at all. I also felt pretty certain that the people at the loan company where she worked wouldn't much appreciate it if she walked in the next day looking like Tina Turner. Instead, I pictured Johnetta looking chic, sophisticated, and feminine.

To begin with, I needed to find a way to elongate Johnetta's round face. I also had to create a style that would show off those incredible eyes. And I had to rejuvenate her hair. Like many black women, Johnetta had used relaxer to straighten her hair. There is nothing wrong with that. But Johnetta had used too much relaxer too often. The result was hair that lay flat on her head without a trace of life or body.

To offset the roundness of her face, the first thing I did was cut Johnetta's hair close to her head on the sides while keeping it as long as possible on the top and at the neck. I also added a couple of fringey bangs to soften her prominent forehead and draw attention to her eyes. In addition, I gave her color a bit of warmth by adding a touch of chestnut to cover the gray. I chose chestnut because it is a dark, rich shade of brown that would blend in nicely with Johnetta's natural hair color. Going with a deep brown shade —rather than, say, ebony—gave Johnetta a softer, less severe look.

It is my opinion that black women should be very careful about coloring their hair. Unless you are a rock star (or want to look like one), it is usually better to make very subtle changes. The reason is simple. When a black woman alters her hair color dramatically, everyone knows it is not real. That's fine if you are in show business or trying to make a statement for some reason. But for most black women using bleach on their hair is rarely appropriate.

That's not to say a black woman can't add richness and warmth to her hair color without looking phony. Look at Johnetta. Even though the change in her color was very subtle, the result is striking. What's more, if you don't go overboard with hair color, it can be a very effective way of adding body. Even before I began styling Johnetta's hair I began to see some signs of life working their way back in.

I would not be telling you the truth if I told you I created this style in five minutes. I explained to Johnetta that the style we chose would take a little longer to do herself. She felt it was worth the extra minutes. I agree.

DOING IT YOURSELF

TOOLS NEEDED: Mousse, blow dryer, large round brush, small round brush, medium-size hot rollers (optional), medium-size curling iron (optional), hair spray.

Johnetta's style is not especially difficult to re-create; it just takes a bit more time. After shampooing, you apply mousse to your roots. Using a large round brush and a blow dryer, you then take one small section of hair at a time and blow it out perfectly straight. (That's the part that takes so much time.) When all your hair is dry, you begin to recurl it by wrapping the ends around a small round brush. I think it is easier to curl Johnetta's kind of hair with a round brush, but if you try this style at home, you may find it easier to use either medium-size hot rollers or a medium-size curling iron. The important thing is to get enough height on top to make your face look longer and narrower.

This particular style may involve a little extra work, but look at the difference it made in Johnetta's appearance. She looked fabulous! I just hope she invites me to her first live concert.

JOHNETTA'S COMMENTS

When I heard that Jose Eber was looking for all kinds of women to make over, I said to myself, What have I got to lose? I knew something had to be done to help me lift my appearance and self-image.

The key to inner beauty, I think, is having inner peace. The way to have inner peace is to be proud of the way you treat other people, to keep yourself healthy, and to work hard at whatever you do. You've got to accept the way you are or do something about changing it. There is nothing worse than a person who complains constantly about a problem and then does nothing to try to fix it.

It is important to try to look your best. It says to the world, "Hey, I care about me—so should you." But a lot of women don't know how to improve themselves or where to go to learn. I wish they could all spend one afternoon with Jose. It really is an uplifting experience. Not because of what he does to your hair, but because of what he does for your spirit.

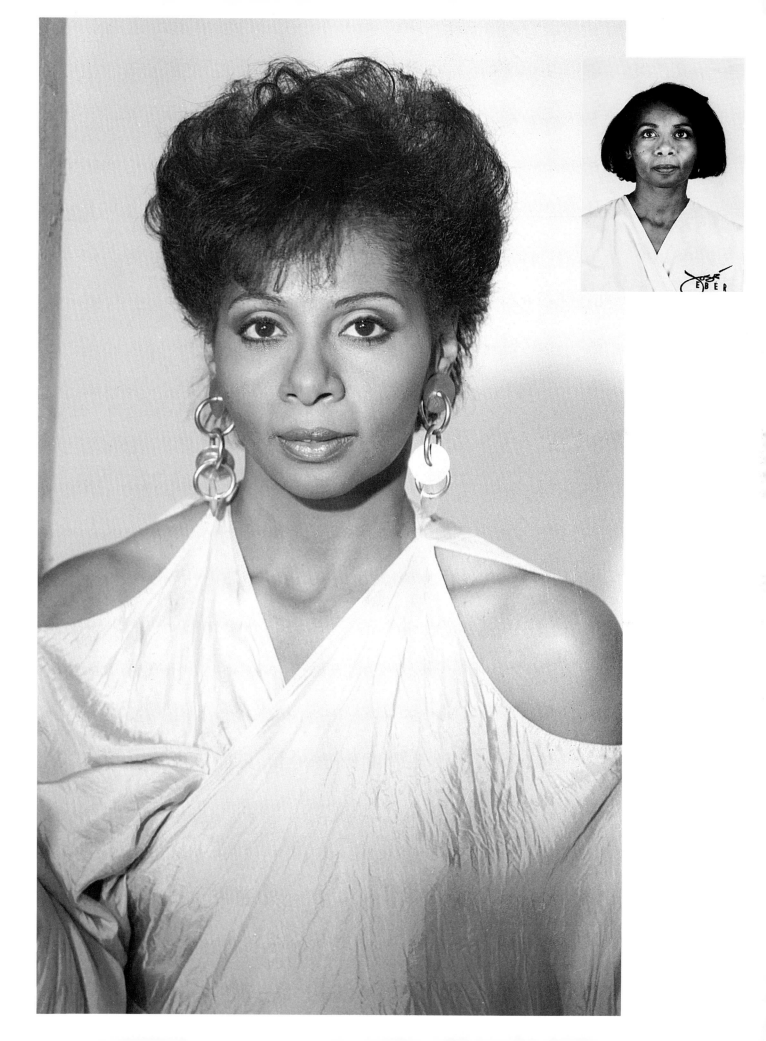

15

BUSINESSLIKE BUT NOT BORING

DANA HENRY

AGE: 42

OCCUPATION: SUPERIOR COURT JUDGE

PROBLEM: THIN, FRIZZY, CURLY HAIR

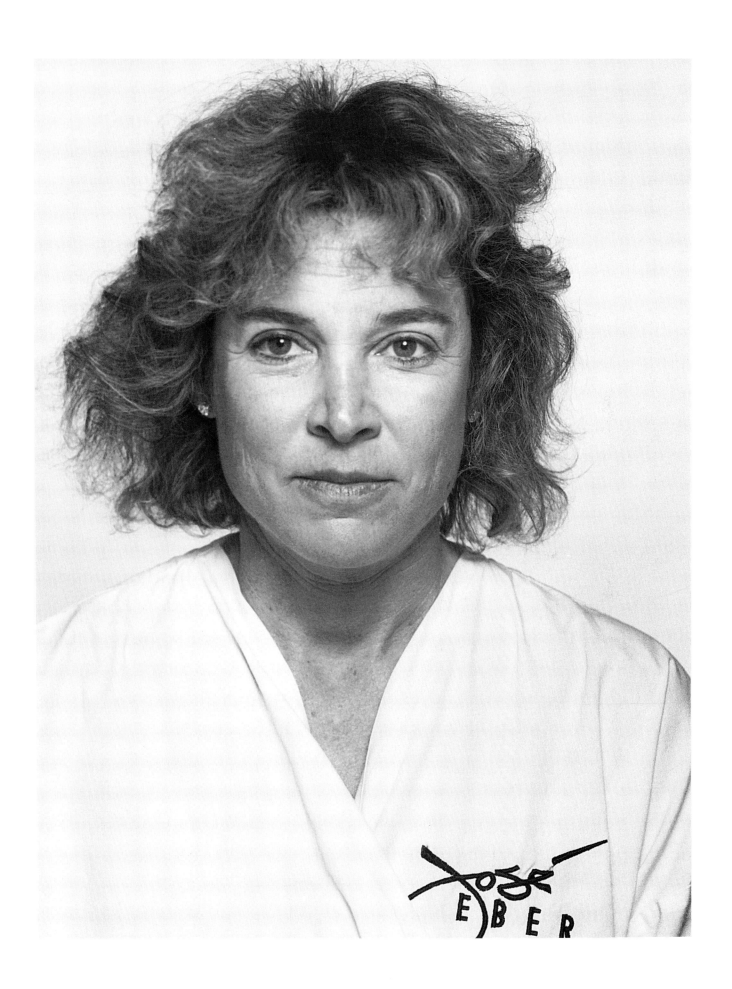

D A N A H E N R Y

Dana Henry is the only woman in this book whom I knew before I started work on it. She had appeared with me on a television show to help me demonstrate that a dedicated professional woman does not have to sacrifice her femininity in order to be taken seriously.

I had been hearing over and over again from women who were pursuing careers as attorneys, accountants, physicians, and so on that they were afraid their credibility would be jeopardized if they came into the office looking *too much* like a woman. That line of thinking struck me as being totally wrong-headed. If a woman feels she is not being treated equally simply because she is a woman, I think she should fight it. By giving up her femininity and trying to look like a man, she is throwing in the towel, succumbing to the notion that women simply don't deserve to be taken seriously as professionals.

When I was introduced to Dana Henry, it occurred to me that she would be the ideal model to demonstrate my point. I mean, who better than a Superior Court judge to demonstrate that a top-notch professional can also be an attractive, feminine-looking woman?

I asked Dana if she would go on TV with me, and she agreed. The show wound up having a huge impact. Its message—that businesslike does not have to be boring—seemed to me important enough to be worth repeating here.

o o o

When I first met Dana, she looked exactly the way one might expect a judge to look—very severe, very conservative, very boring. Dana agreed. She had been going through some big changes in her life and was ready to change her image, too. In a sense, we helped each other. I helped Dana realize she was pretty, and she helped me prove that it was okay to *be* pretty.

The first thing I did to Dana was lighten her hair. Streaking it with a combination of honey, caramel, and golden highlights immediately softened her face and took away the hard edge. The change in hair color also replaced the gray in her complexion with a warm glow. And it loosened her natural curl a bit.

I didn't shorten her hair very much, but I did do a lot more layering to achieve a fuller, more delicate feeling around her face. Dana used to let her hair fall to the sides of her head. I showed her that wearing it back away from her face would give her a richer, more chic look. I also showed her the value of spending a few extra minutes with a round brush and blow dryer taking the kink out of her tight curls and stretching them into more subtle waves. I encourage every woman to look her best, but in Dana's case it was especially important that she look as if every detail mattered. When she let her hair dry naturally, the result wasn't very sophisticated.

What happened to Dana in my chair was amazing. I've never seen a deeper, more obvious change in the spirit. I'm not sure she ever thought of herself as good-looking until that very moment. Like many women, her attention had always gone to her family first, then her career. There was never the time, the desire, or the know-how for personal attention. In Dana's eyes, vanity had no place in the courtroom. I hope I helped her to understand that when you feel good about the way you look, that edge of confidence shows through in every aspect of your life. Of course she won't be sitting in the courtroom thinking about how she looks—she won't have to.

DOING IT YOURSELF

TOOLS NEEDED: Mousse, styling spritz, blow dryer, medium-size round brush, medium-size curling iron (optional), medium-size hot rollers (optional), hair spray.

If you have Dana's type of hair—the kind that is very thin and difficult to work with—you should use both mousse and styling spritz for more control after shampooing. Then section your hair in small pieces, wrap each section around the medium-size round brush, and blow-dry it completely, away from your face. After all your hair has dried in soft curves, take a comb and tease the roots a little bit on top and around your face. This will give you more fullness and height. Then pull a few little bangs down onto your forehead and add the finishing touch of hair spray.

If you are trying this style at home and haven't quite got the hang of using a round brush and blow dryer, the same look can be achieved by using a medium-size curling iron or medium-size hot rollers. Just be sure to brush your hair well after using electrical curling devices to soften the amount of curl you get. The secret to this style is delicate waves. If you come out looking like a French poodle, you'll know you've gone too far.

DANA'S COMMENTS

At the time I was introduced to Jose, many changes were taking place in my life. My career was flourishing, but my personal life was unsteady. Recently divorced, I was just beginning to test the waters, to see how well I could function as a single woman after fifteen years of marriage. My social self-confidence was at an all-time low, and I was desperately searching for positive reinforcements to make the transition smoother. When I was told about Jose and what he needed for his television program, I thought, Hey, this is a great place to start.

What happened after that is difficult to put into words. In what seemed like casual conversation at the time, Jose changed my whole mind-set about the way I saw myself. Throughout my life, I've received a lot of positive recognition in my career and have always felt extremely rewarded as a mother. That was enough for me. Or so I thought. Then I got divorced and realized how long it had been since I had felt like a woman. Not a mother or a judge, just a woman. Jose made me feel feminine again. I can't tell you how exhilarating that was for me. He taught me that looking good doesn't take away from my credibility, it *adds* to it. Simply because I feel better, I am better.

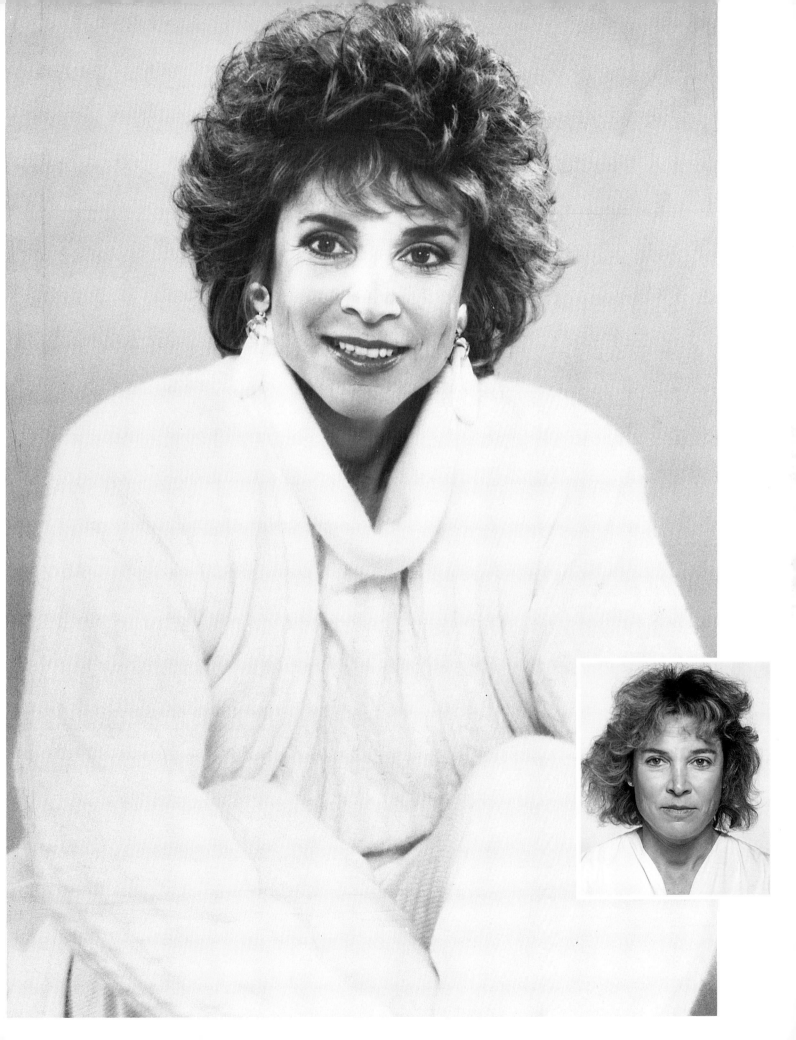

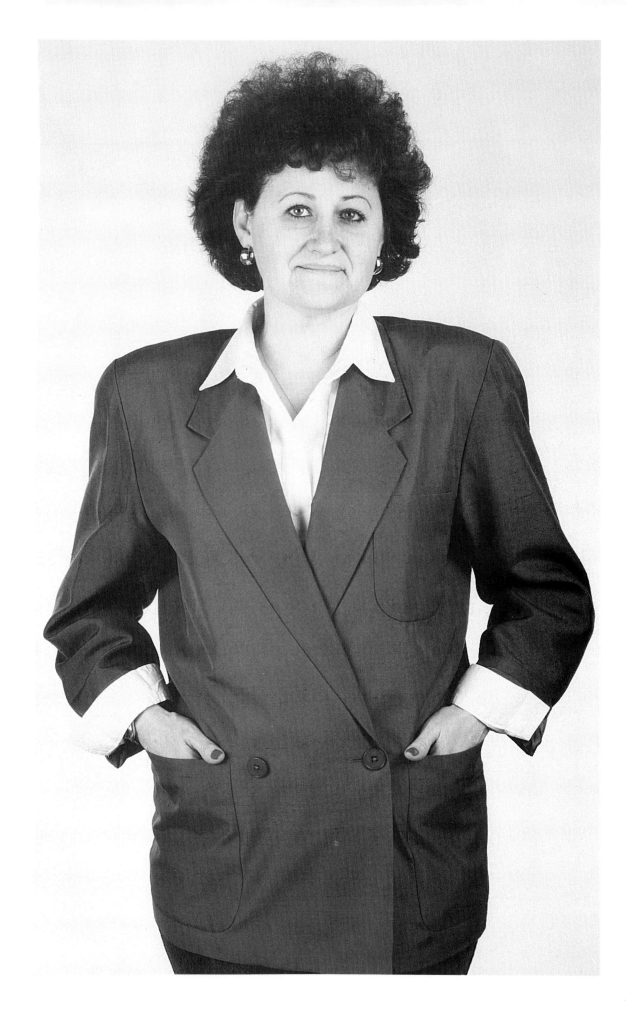

16

"I'LL NEVER BE GORGEOUS"

C. G. O'CONNOR

AGE: 42

OCCUPATION:

PROMOTION AND PUBLIC
RELATIONS DIRECTOR

PROBLEM:

POINTED CHIN;

SHORT CURLY HAIR;

SHARP, ANGULAR FEATURES

C. G. O'CONNOR

The second I saw C. G. I wanted her in my book. Not only did I like her right away, but I knew many women could relate to the things she felt were her problems. She walked right up to me and said what was on her mind: "Look. I've got a pointed chin, a long nose, I wear glasses, and my hair is out of control. I know I'll never be gorgeous, but I have a very visible job and I want to look my best. What can you do about it?"

This was a woman who knew how to get what she wanted. Just as I was going to ask about her life-style, C. G. said, "I work long hours, have a fifteen-year-old son, and I belong to six different community organizations. I'm busy, but I want to learn."

How could I refuse such a dynamic woman? The truth is I couldn't. I really wanted to help. I knew that C. G. had the charm, confidence, and sense of humor to make it no matter what she looked like, but I wanted to make her look the best she ever had in her life. There was something about her personality that reminded me of someone I knew. I couldn't think, at first, whom this little dynamo brought to mind. And then it came to me. Of course, it was the TV talk-show host, Sally Jessy Raphaël. . . .

I looked at C. G. for a long time before I figured out how to help her. I said to myself, What is the first thing you notice about C. G. when you see her face? Because her features are quite angular and her hair was so dark, she looked harsh and stern. But she isn't that way at all, and I didn't want her to appear that way to anyone. So I decided to make her a blonde. C. G. loved the idea. I went with a light strawberry-blond shade because her natural hair color had quite a bit of auburn in it. As soon as we changed the color, the effect was dramatic.

C. G. is a businesswoman. Her work brings her into the public eye regularly, and she is photographed often. She needed a style that was smart, clean, and crisp. With that in mind, I took away all the bushiness on the sides and back, and layered the top. Then I straightened her curl to a soft wave. Bringing some hair onto the forehead softened the lines of her face considerably. By the time I was finished with C. G., she had the look of an attractive, savvy businesswoman. For her part, C. G. was absolutely speechless. Her eyes were twinkling, though, so I knew she was happy.

For C. G. to maintain her new look at home by herself will be easy.

DOING IT YOURSELF

TOOLS NEEDED: Gel, blow dryer, vent brush, hair spray.

The kind of bleach we used on C. G. would soften even the most naturally curly hair. Still, you won't have to worry about using a curling iron or hot rollers. A small dollop of gel (about the size of a quarter in the palm of your hand), worked through your wet hair from the roots to the ends, will give it the little extra weight it needs to keep from frizzing. All you need to do after that is blow-dry your hair away from your face with a vent brush. When it is dry, pull your hair forward with your hands, spray it—and you're ready for anything.

I think C. G. wound up looking fabulous. The important thing, however, is that C. G. thinks she looks fabulous. She told me this experience changed her life; for the first time, ever, she feels confident about the way people see her.

C. G.'S COMMENTS

The reason I went to Jose's salon was to encourage a friend who had been through a rough divorce and was finally ready to get back into the social mainstream. I knew she wouldn't go by herself, so I went along for moral support. Besides, I thought it would be fun to meet Jose Eber. I had heard a lot about him and had seen his work on television for years. I really don't think it occurred to me, at least not as first, that I might be chosen for his book. But all of a sudden, I thought to myself, Hey, I've been through *two* rough divorces, and it's time *I* got back in the social mainstream! I couldn't believe how much I wanted it. I have never thought of myself as pretty, but when Jose walked by me that night I was overcome with hope.

I'm no expert on outer beauty. I grew up listening to my brother tell me that I was ugly enough to stop a freight train. I believed him. But I always had lots of friends as a child, and I always had a boyfriend. When you are not born with good looks, you've got to rely on your personality. This became more and more obvious as I got older. I see it like this—sooner or later everyone's looks fade. It's a fact of life. Those who have depended solely on outer beauty to get by are going to find themselves in bad shape when their looks go. I'm lucky. I developed the communication skills I needed to become successful a long time ago.

I know I'm bright, I know I'm outgoing, I know I can do anything I want to do. I don't mind that I'm not beautiful. Thanks to Jose, I'm attractive. And that's the best I can do. I'm satisfied.

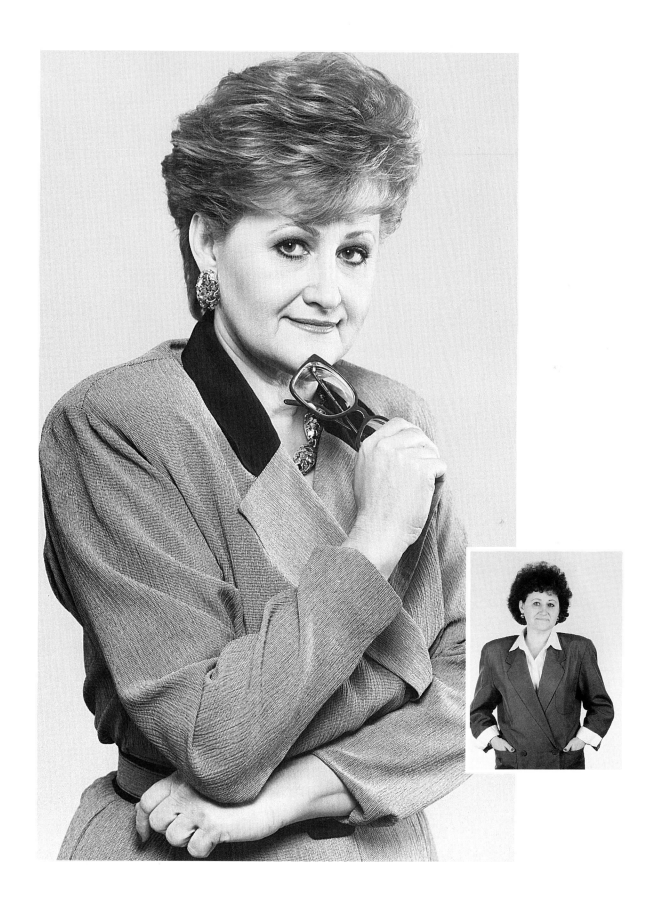

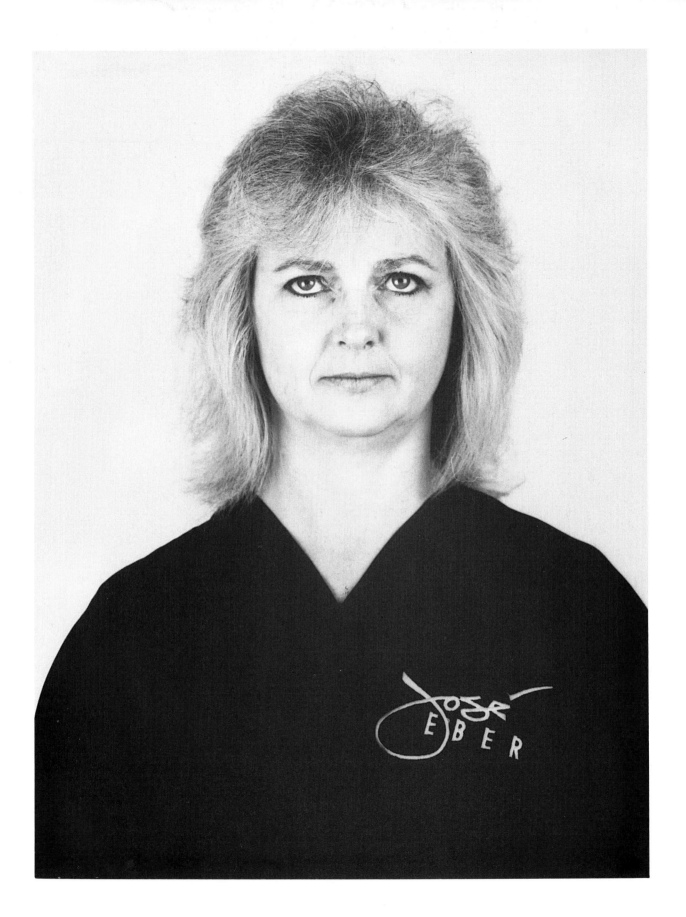

17

A SILVER FOX

D'ANN
FRASCA SNYDER

AGE: 43

OCCUPATION:

EXECUTIVE

ASSISTANT

PROBLEM:

OUTDATED STYLE,

DAMAGED ENDS

D'ANN FRASCA SNYDER

I have never been able to understand why so many women dread the prospect of going gray. Silver and white hair can be terribly impressive—as elegant and stylish as any other color. There is no better proof of that than our current First Lady, Barbara Bush. She has white hair and she's proud of it, as well she should be. She looks terrific.

D'Ann Frasca Snyder feels the same way. D'Ann is the kind of person that people like right away. She's cheerful and happy and filled with positive energy. She has never colored her hair, nor has she ever had any desire to do so.

When she sat down on my chair, D'Ann said she was open to anything. Still, I think she was relieved when I told her that I loved her natural color and had no intention of trying to persuade her to change it. What I wanted to change was her basic style, which was outdated. I also wanted to do something about her dry and split ends.

D'Ann is an adventurous woman. She has worked as a skydiving instructor, a groundskeeper at a gold mine, and a disc jockey. She has a lot of interests and is not afraid to try anything. I admire that. The company she currently works for produces syndicated radio specials. Given all that, I wanted to create a style for her that looked chic yet captured her free spirit.

D'Ann has a pretty face with great structure and high cheekbones. She also has nice flat ears. Thus, I knew I could cut her hair short without a problem. Although I left a little bit of length on top, I cut it really close to her head on the sides and at the bottom.

Not every woman can wear her hair as short as D'Ann. Before I decide to cut a woman's hair this short, I scrutinize her appearance from every angle to make sure her bone structure can stand the bareness. D'Ann had an oval face, high cheekbones, a small straight nose, and huge eyes. I could shave her head completely and she'd still look terrific. However, I decided a simple haircut would do just fine.

Sometimes just the smallest changes produce the most dramatic results. The fact is, not every head of hair needs every treatment. I wish I could shake the hand of the person who first said, *"If it ain't broke, don't fix it."*

If D'Ann thought her hairstyle was easy for me to create, she is going to find it even easier to re-create at home.

DOING IT YOURSELF

TOOLS NEEDED: Mousse, gel, blow dryer, hair spray.

To clean wet hair, simply apply a little mousse to the roots. All you have to do after that is blow your hair dry, lifting the top with your hands for height. Moistening your fingers with a bit of gel, slick the sides to your head and gently pull the bangs forward. A spritz of spray and you look like a million.

D'ANN'S COMMENTS

Next to having my two boys, my makeover was the best thing that ever happened to me. Jose has the ability to put a woman in the everyday world armed with her best weapon—self-confidence.

For some reason, it has never seemed to matter as much if men were good-looking. I have always thought it was because women didn't require that of men. When we are looking for a friend, a business associate, or a lover, there are qualities that rate a lot higher on our priority list. Then why, do you suppose, do we require it in ourselves? Could it be because men have often required it in us?

I have never thought my physical appearance measured up to society's standards. I haven't really been bothered by it because I know I'm a good person. I have the two greatest sons a woman could ask for, dear friends, and enough skills that I won't go hungry. Still, I'd always wondered what it would be like to feel really pretty. Now I know.

The changes that have occurred in my life since my makeover are very obvious to me. Everyone has mentioned it. My boss told me I looked stunning. My friends raved, and acquaintances have told me they love the new image. The real difference, though, has come from strangers. I know I'm being noticed in a crowd or walking down the street. It used to be if my eyes looked into those of a stranger, they were met with a blank stare that said, "I don't know you and that's okay with me." Now, when I look into a stranger's eyes, they smile back at me. It's a great feeling. I'm surprised at how much I like it, how much it matters to me. I know that a pretty face can never take the place of a pretty heart, but for the first time ever, I look as good as I feel inside.

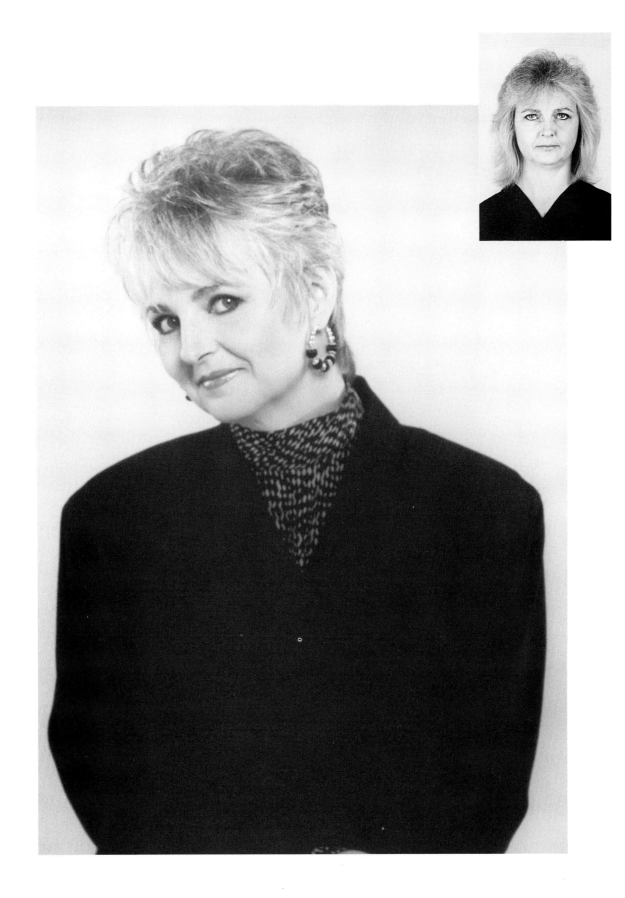

18

GIVING UP A SECURITY BLANKET

LORRAINE
PETTIT

AGE: 44

OCCUPATION:
OWNER,
HOUSEKEEPING
BUSINESS

PROBLEM:
UNFLATTERING
HAIR COLOR,
STYLE, AND LENGTH

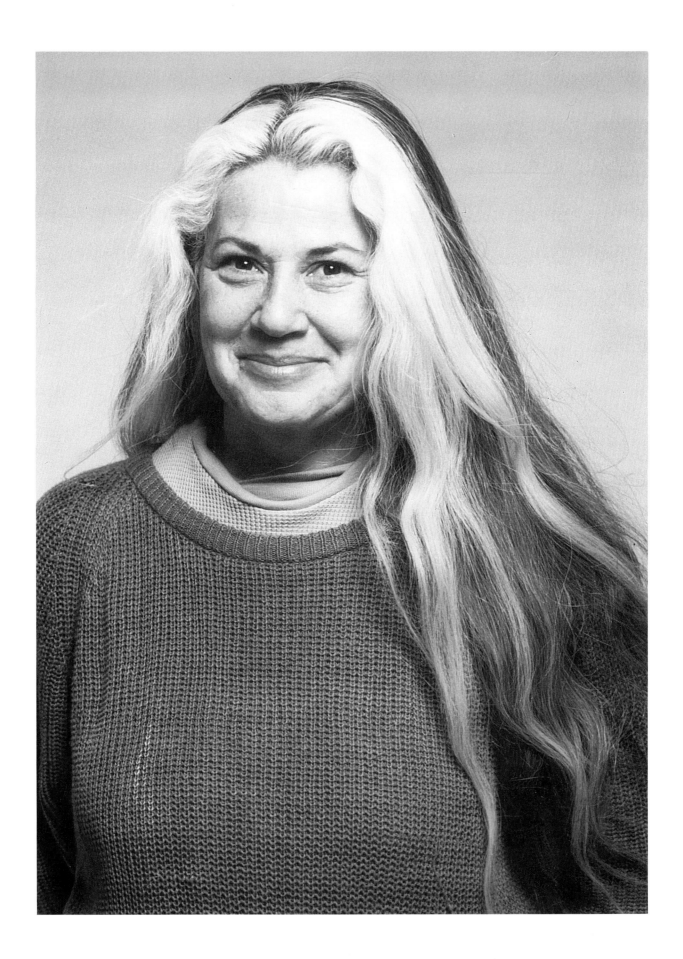

LORRAINE PETTIT

When I met Lorraine, I knew I could do something to help her, but I had no idea the results would be as dramatic as they turned out to be. Though I pride myself in my ability to foresee the finished product when I first look at a woman, the magnitude of Lorraine's hidden beauty shocked me.

Of all the women I met throughout this project, I guess I could relate to Lorraine's fears and nervousness more than anyone else's. For Lorraine, her hair was her security blanket and had been for a very long time. The same is true of me. I have often joked to my friends and family that I must have been Samson in a former life. My hair has always given me a sense of security, even when I was a young boy. Still, when the time comes for me to cut it off, I'll know.

That time had arrived for Lorraine when she came to see me. She said that it had been coming for about three years, and she was finally ready for the big change. She said I could do anything I felt was necessary. She had only one request. Lorraine wanted to save her ponytail in its entirety. In other words, she didn't want me to cut it off an inch at a time. It would be all or nothing. I said no problem. That's not to say that there wasn't a lot of drama when I made the first snip of the scissors. There was.

Lorraine cried, and I felt very badly for her. Not because I thought we had made the wrong decision, but because I knew that for Lorraine losing that hair was like losing a friend.

Lorraine owns a housekeeping business. She works very hard, and as a result her business does very well. Just because she earns her living cleaning other people's homes, there is no reason she should not look as chic and glamorous as any other woman in or out of the business world. Chic comes from inside you. No hairstyle I could give Lorraine could make her look glamorous if she didn't feel that way. But I could tell she had a sense of something untapped inside. I could tell she knew her potential.

Lorraine's hair has a lot of natural body to it. Unfortunately, it had been completely flattened out by the weight of her long tresses. To restore that hidden body, I cut her hair all one length to the chin, giving her a style that was both simple and classic. I had very specific reasons for cutting her hair that particular length. I wanted it long enough so that Lorraine could feel it on the back of her neck and know that she still had hair, yet not so long that she might be tempted to wear it in a ponytail. Old habits die hard, and I was afraid that given the opportunity, Lorraine might revert to her old look before giving the new one a chance.

Because the cut I gave her is one of the classics and not trendy, Lorraine will be able to wear her hair that way forever. That's just as well, for we already know that Lorraine is not a woman to rush into change.

Lorraine's biggest problem was that her hair color looked very unnatural. It didn't have the authenticity of a blend or the drama of a single color. The combination of bleached streaks in front and ash brown in back made her look a lot older than she needed to look. Taken together, her hair seemed gray, and not a pretty gray. I decided to change her color to a honey caramel brown, which would complement her golden skin tone.

Though the new color will require periodic touch-ups (about every six to eight weeks), it turned out to be surprisingly close to Lorraine's natural hue. Sometimes a woman colors her hair for so long that she forgets what her real color actually was.

To my eye, the result was overwhelming. The change in cut and color took ten years off her appearance. Lorraine looked as beautiful on the outside as she is on the inside. And she can go on looking this way with practically no effort at all.

DOING IT YOURSELF

TOOLS NEEDED: Blow dryer, large round brush, hair spray.

Because Lorraine's hair has so much natural body, she doesn't need mousse or styling spritz to re-create this look. The only thing she needs to do is bend the ends of her hair around a large round brush while blow-drying. A squirt or two of hair spray to keep it in place, and that is absolutely it. No fuss, no muss.

LORRAINE'S COMMENTS

I knew I had to do something about my hair. It was as if I had been stuck in a time warp. I just couldn't bring myself to part with it even though I knew I could look a lot better. The experiences, the memories, the security I had in having long hair, were all important to me. Jose understood that. He didn't laugh at my fears, he empathized with them. He talked to me about my career and about my life-style. He kept asking me how I wanted to look. I was afraid he might think that because I make a living cleaning houses, I didn't have the right to be as glamorous as someone who makes her living as a model. After talking with Jose a little more, it became obvious that this was *my* hang-up and not his. He wanted me to look my best, which is what he wants for everyone. I looked around and saw some of the other women whose hair he had styled. Every one of them not only looked beautiful, but felt beautiful as well.

I was ready to feel beautiful, too. I asked Jose to cut my ponytail so I could save it as a memento. The truth is, I thought that if for some reason the cut turned out wrong, I could figure out a way to attach it again like a hairpiece. The rest, as they say, is history. That ponytail will never be used for anything other than a reminder of the incredible experience I had with Jose. I was scared to death while he was cutting it off. I was scared to death while he was styling the hair, and I was scared to death while it was being colored. But when it was all said and done, I don't remember ever feeling more alive. What Jose did for me goes way beyond hair.

When I left the studio on the night of my makeover, I got in my car and took a long drive up the coast. I was too excited to go home, and I wanted some time to think clearly about what had just happened. Was it really a haircut and color change that made me feel so different on the inside? It couldn't be. Then what was it? I began to think about what had happened to me in the three years I'd been wanting to make a change in my appearance. I came up with the idea of starting my own business, and I did it. I worked hard to make it successful, and it is. I set goals, and I achieved them. I have a lot to be proud of. It occurred to me that maybe I wouldn't have looked this good if I hadn't felt this good. Maybe that's the true meaning of beauty.

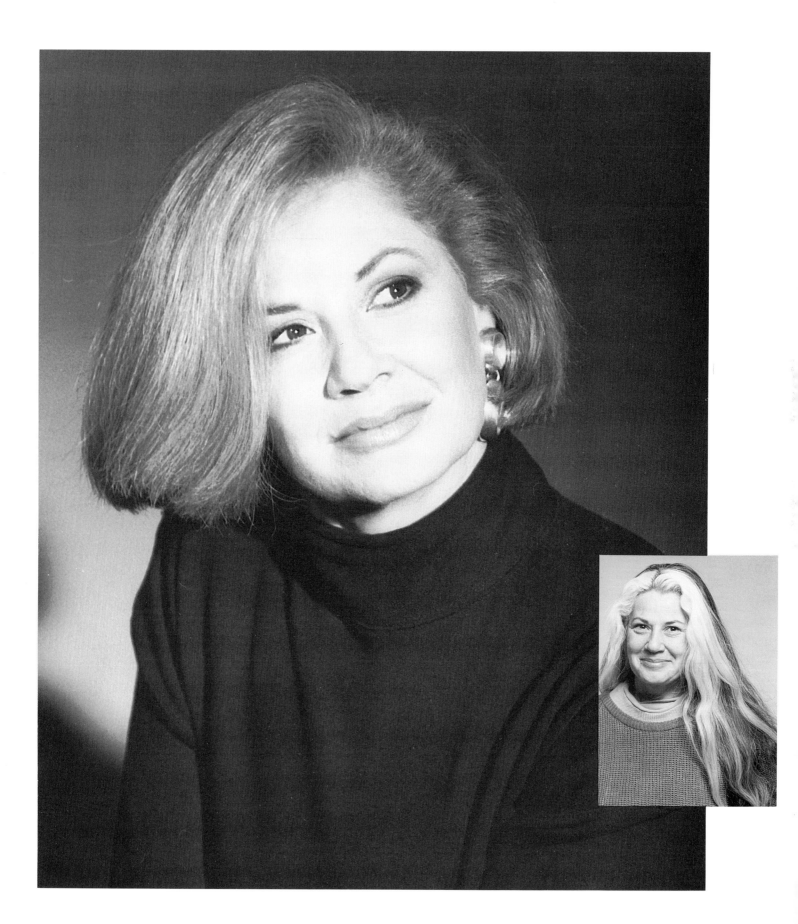

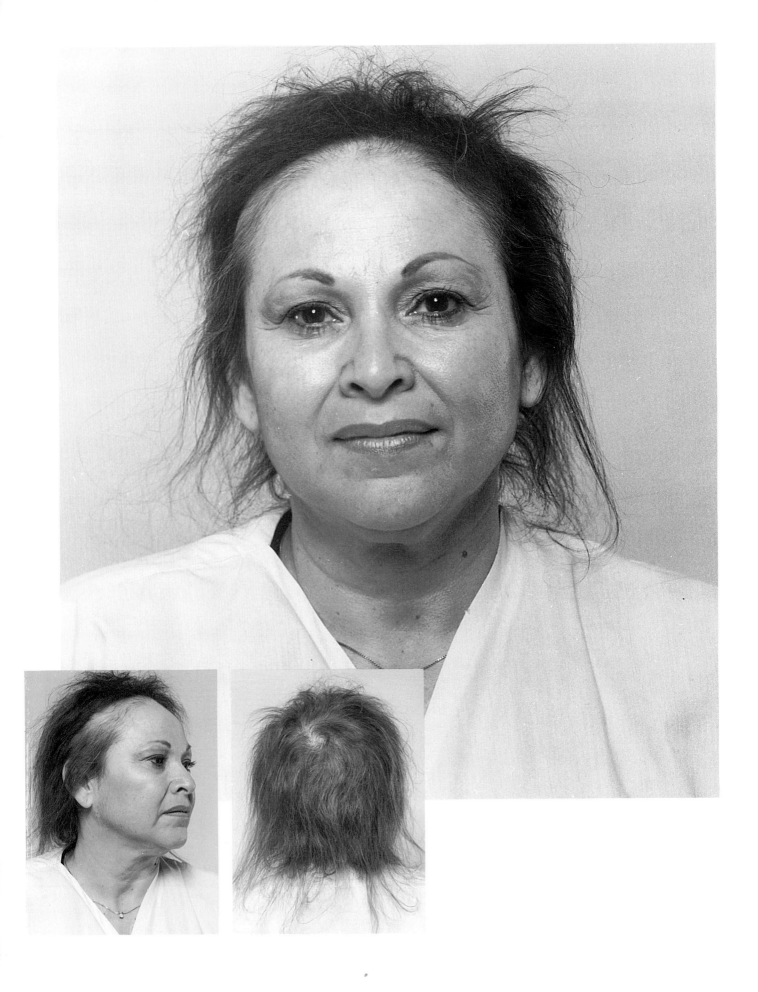

19

AN ALTERNATIVE TO WIGS

SALLY FARVER

AGE: 51

OCCUPATION: WIFE, MOTHER, GRANDMOTHER

PROBLEM: BALDNESS

S A L L Y   F A R V E R

Sally Farver is an exceptional woman with a medical condition that is more common than you might think. When she is under severe stress, her hair falls out. I'm not talking about the kind of stress that comes from getting stuck in traffic or arguing with your boss. I'm talking about the kind of stress that comes from losing your husband to cancer followed by nine operations of your own. Sally's condition is called alopecia areata.

One answer to Sally's problem is to wear a wig. But there is another option, one that I think is better—a hair extension. Hair extensions are pieces of hair sewn directly onto your own hair. They won't work on completely bald men and women, but if you have even a minimal amount of hair, this procedure can be a godsend. It is perfect for cancer patients who have been through chemotherapy and are anxiously waiting for their own hair to grow back.

What makes a hair extension better than a wig is that a hair extension doesn't come off. You can shower, swim, dance, play sports, do anything you want, and you'll be safe.

As a result, hair extensions have become very popular among rock stars and other people in the entertainment business over the last few years. In a matter of hours, a man or woman can have thick, long, natural-looking hair. It is quite remarkable. Of course, it is also a very expensive procedure, so I don't often recommend it merely for cosmetic purposes.

Still, for cancer patients and those with stress-related hair loss, there is no price too high for regaining self-dignity. Many reputable men and women do this procedure, but I have been especially impressed by the work done by a man named Piny Benzaken.

PINY ON SALLY

Sally's problem is fairly typical of the women who come into my office. Sally came to me twelve years ago with her hair looking about the same as it does in her "before" photo. She had lost all her hair during the illness of her first husband. It started to grow back but never finished. She had been wearing a wig up until that point. Sally heard about my hair extensions for men and wondered if I could help her. I knew I could.

I begin by hand-stitching a very thin braid directly to the remaining hair left on the back of the scalp. The braid goes from one side of the head to the other and is firmly woven to the client's natural hair. To that tiny braid I will sew a row of hair extensions. Hair extensions are individual strands of perfectly matched human hair bound together with the strongest nylon.

If the client's hair is not too thin, or if he or she is only interested in adding length (as opposed to thickness), sometimes one row of hair extensions is enough. In Sally's case it wasn't. Her head requires a full weave. I added two more braids and two more rows of extensions before starting on the top.

Adding hair extensions to the top of the head is even more delicate than adding to the back. It is imperative that the braids be so tiny that they are impossible to see. One of the advantages of spending the time and money on hair extensions is that they can look completely natural. If you can see the braids, the procedure is worthless. But when the procedure is done correctly, it's as natural-looking as your own hair. Once you have had hair extensions added and you are happy with the results, it is both a time and a financial commitment. As your hair grows out, the extensions move away from your head and must be tightened regularly.

Just as every hairdresser charges differently for his or her work, the price of hair extensions also varies, depending on the quality of the hair and the quality of the craftsmanship. You can expect to pay approximately $475 to $775 for two rows of braids in the back. To have them tightened, which you'll need done every four to five weeks, the cost is about $85. For a full weave, you can expect to pay anywhere from $1,275 to $1,700 for the initial visit and $115 to $135 for maintenance.

Once your hair extensions are in place, you can treat them just like your own hair. You can cut them, color them, perm them, and wash them without a problem.

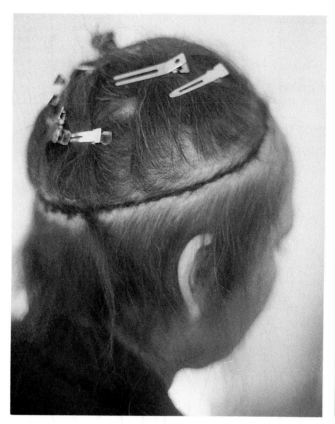
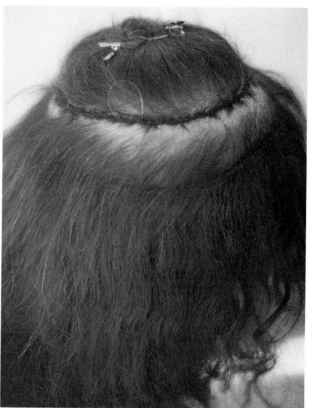
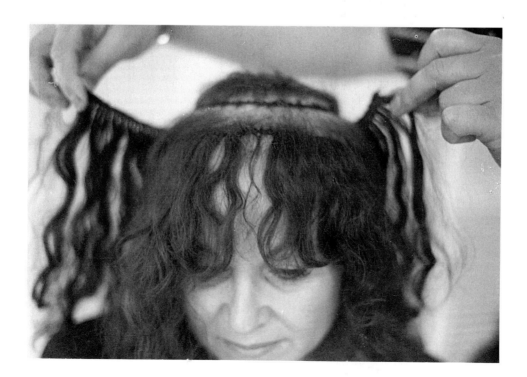

SALLY'S COMMENTS

Hair extensions saved my life. Before I had them, I was nervous every time I went out the front door. If I walked into a party, I was sure everyone was either laughing at me or feeling sorry for me. And frankly I don't know which was worse. If there was even the slightest breeze in the air, I panicked that my wig would blow away, never to be seen again. To be honest, I was better off staying home, so that's just what I did. Although my second husband, Don, never said a word, I know he had to have been frustrated with me. But then we heard about Piny.

He was an answer to a prayer. Today, my life is full. I'm hardly ever home because there is so much I want to enjoy and experience in life. Maybe I'm making up for lost time, but I don't care. I'm having a ball!

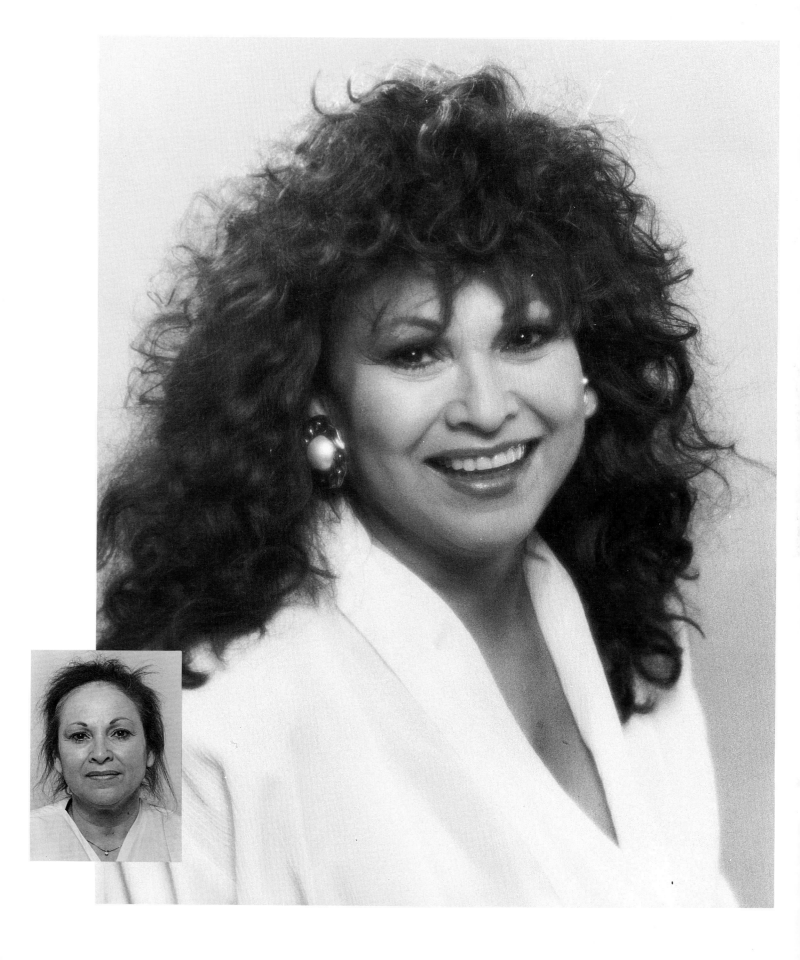

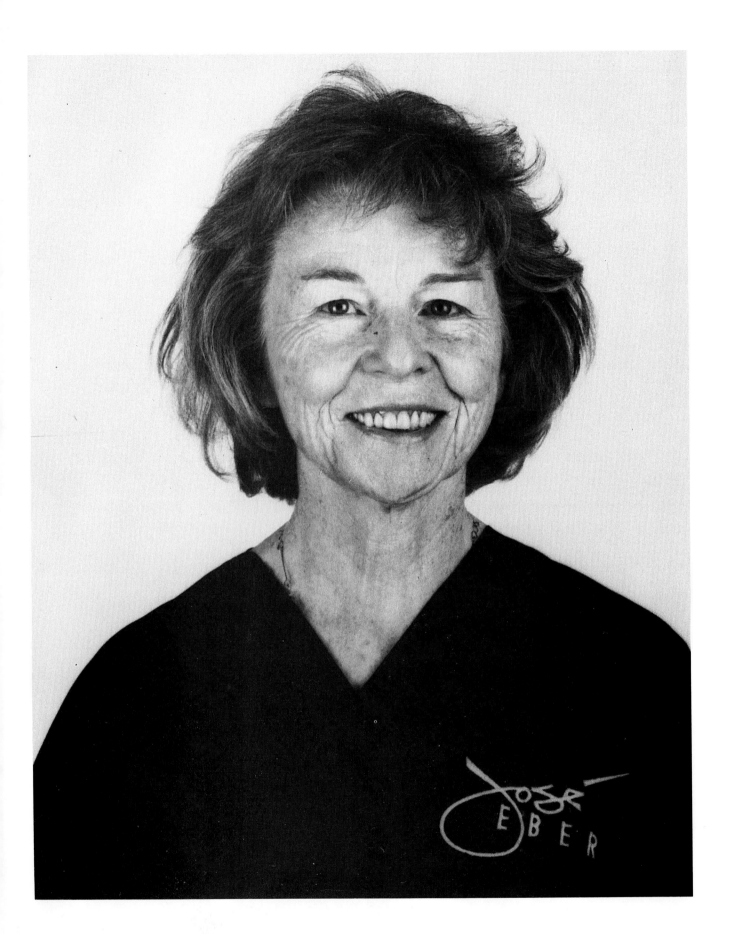

20

OVERCOMING AGE

CARO JONES

AGE: 61

OCCUPATION:
CASTING DIRECTOR

PROBLEM:
THIN, LIFELESS
HAIR;
WRONG COLOR

C A R O   J O N E S

Although Caro is the oldest woman in this book, her spirit is young and vibrant. This was obvious to me at our first meeting. She is bright, witty, and self-confident. She didn't worry about the way she looked, not because she didn't care, but because she didn't think about it. Caro runs a very successful business in Los Angeles, and her days are filled with interest and meaning. She's got more on her mind than hair spray and lipstick.

Caro never felt she had to be beautiful in order to be accepted, either in her personal life or in her professional life. After all, that's not the way *she* determines her friends and business associates. Still, Caro always thought that someday, if she could make the time, it might be fun to have a complete makeover.

The fun thing about consulting with Caro was that she had the greatest attitude. She wasn't nervous about what I might do—anything was fine. Caro just wanted to look better. She had no high expectations or preconceived notions. For some reason, that made me want to thrill her. . . .

The first thing I noticed about Caro was that her hair didn't really have any particular style. It was just sort of there—without body or life. Her hair is very thin, and it had been cut in many layers, making it look even thinner. Because Caro is a very tiny, petite woman, she needs a hairstyle with lots of fullness at the sides. To accomplish that, I cut her hair blunt at the bottom and cleaned up the layers at the sides. The result lent her whole appearance more authority and power.

You can see in Caro's "before" picture that there was very little difference between her ash-blond hair color and her skin tone. The ash not only made her hair look dirty gray, it made her skin look gray as well. In order to look good with ash-brown or ash-blond hair, you've got to have a lot of pink in your skin tone. To be perfectly honest, I don't particularly care for ash on anyone. Given a choice, I'd always opt for the warmer shades of nature. To me, ash looks like what it was named after—ashes.

I replaced Caro's unflattering ash-blond color with a chestnut-and-auburn mixture that made Caro's complexion look much brighter and healthier. At once we saw a sparkle and vitality in Caro that hadn't been evident before.

There was only one catch to Caro's new look. Caro told me that she was used to spending almost no time on herself in the morning. I had to tell her that in order to re-create her new look at home, she would have to work a few extra minutes into her regular morning routine. Her hairstyle requires a little bit of attention.

DOING IT YOURSELF

TOOLS NEEDED: Mousse, styling spritz, blow dryer, medium-size round brush, medium-size curling iron, hair spray.

If your hair is as thin and fine as Caro's, the first thing you must do in order to get style and body is to add either mousse or styling spritz (or maybe both) to the roots after shampooing. Then tip your head down and, using a medium-size round brush, blow your hair completely dry. After that, use the medium-size curling iron to curl the top and the sides away from your face, carefully curling small sections at a time. With your fingers, tug gently on the curls to make sure they're not too tight. Before finishing with hair spray, run the round brush through your hair one more time and pull a few bangs down on your forehead.

CARO'S COMMENTS

Quite frankly, it was an eye-opening experience to see people's reactions to my new look. I have never received so many personal compliments in my life. Everyone mentions it, and truthfully, I feel fantastic. I can honestly say that my business has never been better. I'm sure I'm not doing anything different professionally, but I am also just as sure that my increase in business is a direct result of my positive self-image. I don't think I had a negative self-image before. I'm afraid I had no self-image at all.

I guess it really does make a difference. People, at least strangers, won't take the time to discover inner beauty if the outer beauty isn't there. I'm not talking about physical perfection, but you have to show you care about yourself. If you don't, why should anyone else?

They say the way you look on the outside should be a direct reflection of how you feel on the inside. That sounds pretty good, but what if you're having a horrible day? Should you run into the ladies' room and mess up your hair or take off your makeup? No, I think a better way to say it is that the way you look on the outside should be a direct reflection of how you *want* to feel on the inside.

I want to feel successful, I want to feel loved, and I want to feel attractive. And now, for the first time, I know how to achieve it.

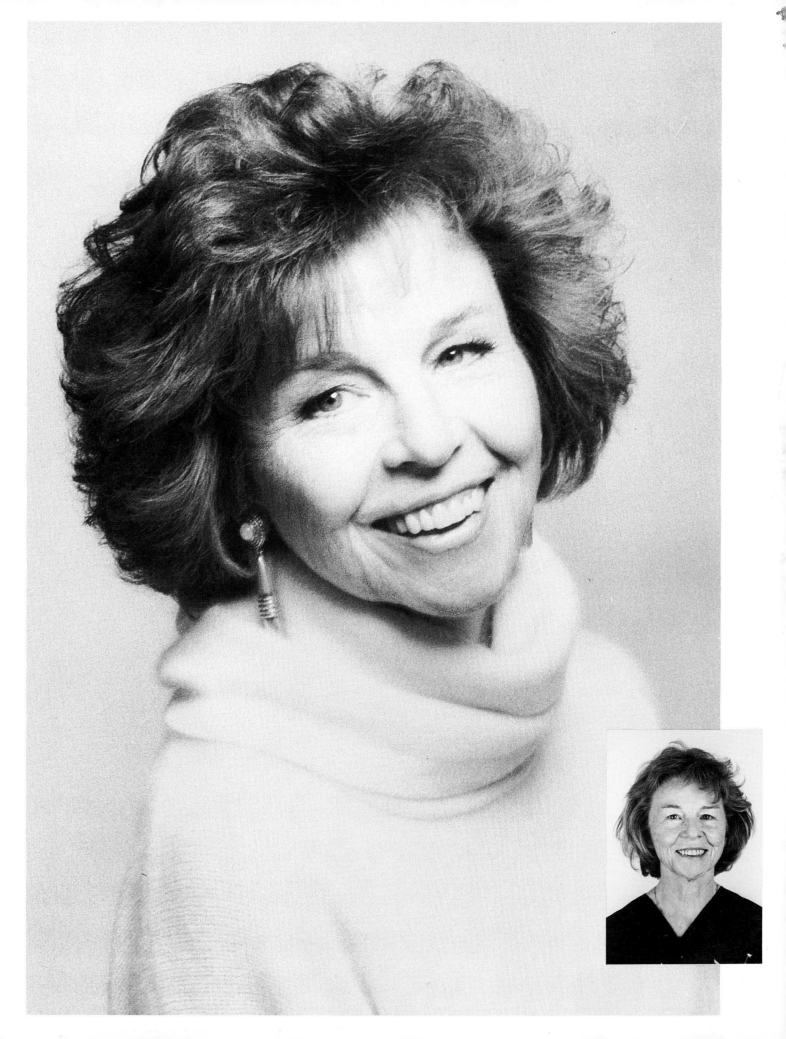

IN CLOSING

Well, now that you have met my new friends, don't you agree that they're beautiful? I hope you enjoyed watching the transformations. I also hope we solved some of your problems along with theirs.

I want each of you to realize and appreciate your own beauty. Remember, the length of your nose, the size of your hips, or the style of your hair doesn't determine how beautiful you are. Your beauty is measured in two ways—how much you love and how much you are loved by others. By now, you must know that it is impossible to be loved by anyone until you love yourself. Remember that you, alone, must face yourself every day. If you look in the mirror and don't see anything you like, a little more styling mousse isn't going to change that. Believe me. If you look in the mirror and don't see anything you like—*go out and do something likable.* That will help you a lot more than changing your hair color. The old saying still holds true. *Pretty is as pretty does.*

On the other hand, if you make an honest effort to be a good person, you can't always worry about what others think. To paraphrase Abraham Lincoln: *You can please all of the people some of the time and some of the people all of the time, but you can't please all of the people all of the time.* It just isn't possible. Sometimes situations occur, for whatever reason, in which you are the only one who believes you are right. When this happens you must first be willing to look at the situation objectively and reevaluate your opinion. If you still believe you are right—stick to your guns! There is a great deal of pride to be taken in such self-confidence. (There is also a great deal of strength to be found in admitting you are wrong and apologizing—when necessary.)

What does all of this have to do with beauty? Everything. If you have inner beauty, it is much easier to find outer beauty. When you see yourself through gentler eyes, you'll see the whole world through gentler eyes. You will be able to look at what you once thought was a flaw and understand that it is a personal distinction. You will have the ability to correct the things you can and accept the things you can't. With a smile. You'll take pride in both your internal and external appearance. Maybe you'll even treat yourself to a makeover. I would be flattered to think I may have motivated you into doing something kind for yourself. Writing this book certainly motivated me into doing something kind for *myself.* After forty years of never having a regular or serious exercise routine, I finally decided it was time I got myself into good shape. As a result, I called on the expertise of personal trainer Rick Clark. (Though I wanted to do this for myself, I also wanted to do it safely and wisely.) Rick has put me on a workout schedule that is strenuous yet within my capabilities. Every week I feel stronger and healthier, and I know I'm doing something to make me more likable—to me!

I told you at the beginning that if you took care of your inner beauty, I would help you with your outer beauty. Perhaps this book has given you some new ideas on both. Maybe you'll even pick it up again when you're having a down day and feel a little better. I would like that.

Thank you for giving me the opportunity to introduce you to my friends. Remember, they only looked beautiful at the end because they were beautiful in the beginning. Learning how to make the most of themselves was not difficult. You can do it, too.

AUTHOR'S NOTE

Like the women you have found throughout the book, the two women who appear with me on the cover are not professional models.

Brogan Bertrand is thirty-nine years old and works as a promotion manager for Weider Publications. As you can see in her "before" picture, her hair was very damaged from a series of bad perms. Still, she was quite reluctant to have it cut short for fear of having what she referred to as "middle-aged hair." Looking youthful is a desire of many women, but for Brogan it is especially important because she has a boyfriend twelve years her junior. I assured Brogan we could give her a younger, fresher look if we got rid of the damage. She agreed to let me try, but I must tell you the truth: as her hair fell to the floor, tears fell from her eyes. To Brogan, long hair was a symbol of youth, and she saw it disappearing right in front of her. I was sympathetic to her feelings, although I could picture the end results looking absolutely fantastic. She has gorgeous high cheekbones and a well-defined jawline, and I knew that getting rid of that frizz would truly show off her natural beauty. Although you cannot see it in her black-and-white "before" picture, Brogan also had remnants of an old, artificial-looking color job, which added to the problem. I took her back to her natural color, a beautiful chestnut brown. Look at her now. Brogan looks a good ten years younger than when we started. Believe me when I tell you that that smile you see on her face now is very much the real thing.

Perri Cline is thirty-one years old and works as a management systems specialist for Hughes Aircraft Company. Her hair was basically in good condition, but it was flat and lifeless without any particular style. I decided to give her a spiral perm, which would accomplish two positive results. The chemical reaction of any type of permanent on the hair will automatically lighten it a few shades. I didn't want to dramatically change Perri's color because I think she looks terrific as a blonde. I just wanted to give her some pizzazz and excitement. The small change in color she got from the perm was just enough. A spiral perm (which we discussed at greater length in the book) gives the hair a tremendous amount of body without a tight curl. This perm will last Perri approximately three months and require virtually no effort whatsoever to maintain. She is an avid athlete and usually spends her free afternoons bicycling up and down the coast with her husband Terry. The less amount of time spent fiddling with her hair, the happier she is. Other than a bit of reshaping and a slight trim of the ends we didn't change the length of her hair at all. This was such a simple procedure, but as you can see her hair went from flat to fabulous.

I would like to extend a special thank you to the very talented Jeremy Mariage for his help in creating these great cover hairstyles, and my friend and makeup artist extraordinaire, Darren Lazenby, for the fabulous finishing touches he lent to the cover.